HEADACHE RELIEF

A Comprehensive, Up-to-Date,

Medically Proven Program

That Can Control and Ease Headache Pain

Alan M. Rapoport, M.D.,
and
Fred D. Sheftell, M.D.

FOUNDERS AND DIRECTORS,
THE NEW ENGLAND CENTER FOR HEADACHE,
STAMFORD, CONNECTICUT

A Fireside Book
Published by SIMON & SCHUSTER
NEW YORK   LONDON   TORONTO   SYDNEY   TOKYO   SINGAPORE

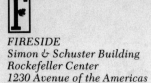

FIRESIDE
Simon & Schuster Building
Rockefeller Center
1230 Avenue of the Americas
New York, New York 10020

First Fireside Edition 1991

FIRESIDE and colophon are
registered trademarks of Simon & Schuster Inc.

Designed by Edith Fowler
Manufactured in the United States of America

10 9 8 7 6 5 4 3 2 1
10   (pbk)

Library of Congress Cataloging in Publication Data

Rapoport, Alan M.
    Headache relief: a comprehensive, up-to-date, medically
proven program that can control and ease headache pain/
Alan M. Rapoport and Fred D. Sheftell.
        p. cm.
    Includes index.
    1. Headache—Popular works.   I. Sheftell, Fred
D.   II. Title.
    [DNLM: 1. Exercise Therapy.   2. Headache—
diet therapy.   3. Headache—drug therapy.
4. Headache—etiology.   WL 342 R219h]
RB128.R37   1990
616.8'491—dc20
DNLM/DLC
for Library of Congress   90-10049
ISBN 0-671-70065-0   CIP
ISBN 0-671-74803-3 (pbk)

We would like to dedicate this work to our wives, our children, our patients, and our colleagues who encouraged us to start The New England Center for Headache. Without their advice and support we might never have embarked on our journey . . .

ALAN M. RAPOPORT
FRED D. SHEFTELL

ACKNOWLEDGMENTS

We would like to thank all those who helped to develop and write this book: especially Betsy Ryan, president of Bascom Communications, Rachel Kranz, and our colleagues at The New England Center for Headache. We have greatly appreciated the support of our editor, Bob Bender. Thanks go also to the pioneers of headache research and treatment in this country and Europe, especially the late John Graham. Thanks go to Lee Kudrow who encouraged us from the start and who has always been there for us, guiding us and making it all possible. Thanks to The Greenwich Hospital Association for its belief in us and its groundbreaking work in the treatment of headache.

CONTENTS

INTRODUCTION

HEADACHE: A GENUINE DISORDER

OVER THE MANY YEARS we have worked with headache patients, we've been struck by one thing above all: the extent to which headache patients want to be listened to, understood, and believed. Most of our patients have been suffering from headaches for years. They have usually had frustrating experiences with earlier efforts to treat their condition. They come to us with many doubts about health professionals—and about themselves. They often feel isolated, abandoned, and guilty.

In large part, we feel their responses have to do with a general feeling among the public—and among some members of the medical community—that headache is not a genuine disorder. To someone who has not experienced it, the pain of headache may seem trivial, not worthy of serious consideration. To health professionals not aware of the latest literature, headache may seem a minor ailment that reflects nothing more serious than a stressful day or, at worst, a Type A personality who needs to learn to relax.

Headache sufferers themselves may have absorbed this view, and consequently do not understand why this seemingly trivial problem continues to radically disrupt their lives. They may feel guilty about "making too much" of their headache pain, or ashamed of not being able to prevent the disorder.

We, on the other hand, assert that headache is a valid medical disorder—as genuine a medical problem as diabetes, hypertension, or heart disease. Research, particularly that of the last ten years, has begun to demonstrate that the sources of chronic or severe headache are neither a tense personality nor a stressful day, but rather a set of biochemical reactions within the brain.

Unfortunately, these mechanisms don't show up in x-rays, in blood tests, or in any other common medical procedure. Unlike the pain of ulcers or colitis, the pain caused by headache has no easily visible source. This reflects more on the current state of medical knowledge than on the reality of the condition, however. Just as we now distinguish between the cramps caused by ulcers and the occasional discomfort of indigestion, so must we come to recognize the difference between the chronic condition of migraine, cluster, or muscle-contraction headaches and the occasional head pain that can be relieved by a single dose of aspirin.

THE HEADACHE MECHANISM AND ITS TRIGGERS

The basic premise of our philosophy, then, is that *headache has its source in a biological mechanism,* apparently one that the headache sufferer is born with (Chapter 2). Once that mechanism is in place, however, many different factors may set it off. It is the variety and frequent unpredictability of these headache *triggers* that leads to much of the confusion about what *causes* headache.

These triggers may act alone or in combination, which adds further to the confusion. For example, one common headache trigger involves female hormones—hence the pattern among many women of menstrual migraines, or migraines that take place only before or after the onset of menopause. Another common trigger is certain types of food (Chapter 7), for example, refined sugar, or the tyramine found in some cheeses. For some women, either trigger is sufficient to set off a migraine. For others, each trigger works only in combination: e.g., a woman may get a headache from eating sugar, but only around the time of her period.

Different types of headaches have different triggers, which are discussed in more detail in Chapter 2. However, generally speaking, the most common triggers include the following: hormones, diet, changes (such as changes in weather or the season, traveling through time zones, skipping a meal, altering a schedule, etc.), and sensory stimuli (such as flickering lights, some odors, strong sunlight, etc.). Psychological factors, such as personality issues, stress, and family systems, may also act as headache triggers. It is the role of these factors, of course, which has been the source of the greatest confusion about the causes of headache.

THE ROLE OF PSYCHOLOGICAL FACTORS

Because of the great confusion surrounding this issue, our outlook bears repeating: *Psychological factors are not, in most cases, the ultimate cause of chronic headaches.* However, psychological factors may act as triggers that *set off* the basic biological mechanism that the headache sufferer is born with.

For many years, doctors and other health professionals assumed that people with headache suffered from some type of psychological or character weakness that made them especially vulnerable to headaches. Medical literature spoke of the "migraine personality": the driven, perfectionistic, self-critical person who was prone to make unrealistic demands on self and others.

We now understand that there is no such thing as a migraine personality. That is, such a personality may exist, but it has no statistical significance in relation to migraine. Many people with the so-called migraine personality do not suffer from migraine; many people without that personality do suffer from migraine or from some other form of chronic headache.

Of course, if a person does have a demanding or self-critical personality *and* a biological tendency to headache, the personality may generate occasions for stress which in turn trigger the pre-existing biological mechanism. Thus, although the personality doesn't cause the headaches, it may help to produce occasions that set them off.

However, personality and environmental stress factors play a role in all sorts of diseases. Diabetes, for example, is commonly accepted as a physical disorder of the pancreas that produces a shortage of insulin. Few would argue that there is a diabetic personality, or that this personality in some way causes the pancreas to malfunction. On the other hand, during times of physical or emotional stress, diabetics frequently need to change their dosage of insulin. Personality and environmental factors play a role in how diabetics are affected by their condition, even though they do not create the condition.

Similarly, people with the biological condition that creates chronic headaches may be affected by personality and environmental factors. They may also be affected by diet, changes in weather, and other nonpsychological factors. The patient and the health professional who attribute everything to psychological causes may be misdiagnosing one or more headache triggers. Something that has been attributed to a tense personality may be corrected by a simple change in diet—but this opportunity for improvement will be missed if all headaches are assumed to be psychological in origin.

On the other hand, once the biological mechanism for headache has been set off, the pattern of getting a headache sometimes takes on a life of its own. We see this most clearly with children. If parents reward their child for having headaches by giving them special privileges or allowing them to avoid difficult situations, the parents are helping to reinforce a pattern that increases the chance of more frequent headaches.

Also, if an adult feels free to say "no" or to ask for help only when he or she has a headache, that adult is reinforcing the likelihood of getting headaches more often. This doesn't mean that psychological factors are the ultimate *cause* of the headache, but it does mean that psychological triggers are operating actively. In such a case, the child or the adult may need to focus on psychological approaches as well as on any physical treatment that may be prescribed.

THE ROLE OF MEDICATION

Since headache is a biologically based condition, it may be appropriate to treat it with medication, as well as in other ways. As we discuss at length in Chapter 3, headache medication may be preventive or symptomatic. Preventive medication is taken daily, with the goal of reducing the likelihood that a headache will be triggered. Symptomatic medication is taken when an actual headache is beginning, with the goal of preventing the headache from continuing.

The doctor who is prescribing medication should be sure to explain the proper procedure for taking the medication, as well as the goals of treatment, the medicine's effects, and its possible side effects. The long-term goal for any prescription of headache medication is to reduce the dosage as much as possible, or to eliminate the medication entirely, once the biological mechanisms have quieted or have resolved themselves (Chapters 5 and 6).

Frequently, nonmedication therapy may be used along with medication, increasing the effectiveness of both. Patients may also use medication as a means to control headache while they're learning how to use nonmedication therapies. When the nonmedication therapies are being used effectively, the medication may be reduced or dropped entirely, under the doctor's supervision.

The strongest and most effective headache medications need to be prescribed. However, many patients come to us with a history of taking off-the-shelf medication for headache relief. Frequently, these patients are taking multiple doses of nonprescription pain relievers several times a week, or even every day. As we explain in Chapter 3, this overuse of medication may actually increase the patient's chance of getting frequent headaches, in what is known as the "rebound effect." Anyone who is taking nonprescription pain relievers more often than once or twice a week should consult a health professional to determine other ways of treating chronic headache.

Similarly, patients who are taking symptomatic medication should be sure to stay in close contact with their doctors. If symptomatic medication of any kind is overused, it may produce more frequent headaches, due to the rebound effect. Patients should continue to discuss this possibility with their doctors—and should certainly never take more than the prescribed dose or receive prescriptions from more than one doctor. Your doctor should always be aware of how much medication you are taking.

WORKING WITH YOUR HEALTH PROFESSIONAL

Clearly, for headache treatment to be effective, both health professional and patient must be willing to work together in a cooperative, collaborative relationship. Each person must be willing to be honest with the other, and to respond to the other person's suggestions.

In our view, the health professional's responsibility is to be honest and clear about the goals of treatment, to fully explain the pros and cons of any form of treatment that is suggested, to compare the proposed treatment to other possibilities, and to listen respectfully to the patient's response. The health professional should also continue to monitor the effect of the treatment, and to be willing to change the treatment based on its actual role in the patient's life. Finally, the health professional should be reasonably available to answer questions and respond to possible difficulties that arise in any course of treatment.

The patient, on the other hand, is responsible for being fully honest with the health professional, particularly about his or her behavior with medication. The patient should be sure to be fully informed about any treatment that's being proposed, and, once he or she has agreed to treatment, to follow the doctor's suggestions fully and cooperatively. The patient is responsible for being aware of how the treatment is affecting him or her, and of reporting these effects to whoever is supervising the treatment.

Patients may also need to recognize that full treatment of their headaches may involve changes in diet, exercise, life-style, and the like. While health professionals may offer some support for these changes, the patient is also responsible for finding the necessary support. The patient who continues to drink or who fails to exercise, despite the doctor's explanation of how this increases the likelihood of headache, cannot then expect the doctor simply to prescribe higher doses of pain relievers. Patients who are unwilling to look at the psychological role of headaches must recognize that they may be interfering with their own treatment.

Finally, patients must have a realistic idea of how much they can expect from their doctors. As we continue to stress, the ultimate source of headache is in a biological condition, a condition for which at the present time there is no cure. That means that headaches may be controlled, but not cured. Thus patients may be able to go for long periods of time without needing medication—but then suddenly, for some reason, find that the biological mechanism has been set off again. Thus treatment must be renewed and possibly altered. Understanding the nature of headache and its treatment helps to make clear that the renewed onset of headache is not a "defeat," but merely a recurrence of a chronic, intermittent condition that must be coped with.

WHAT THE FUTURE HOLDS

We believe that the future looks much brighter for those who suffer from headaches. There is increasing interest by scientists and researchers throughout the world in clarifying the mechanisms that produce head pain. These discoveries will lead in turn to new headache treatment, both with and without medication.

Most of the current research involves the biology of serotonin and its receptors. Serotonin, as we explain in Chapter 2, is a neurotransmitter, one of the chemicals in the brain that is used to transmit information. Serotonin research is providing new insight into depression, schizophrenia, and sleep disorders, as well as into all varieties of headache. It appears to promise exciting new developments in our ability to understand and treat headache pain.

Besides increased research, increased education should raise the level of understanding among the medical community and the general public. As headache comes to be accepted as a genuine biological disorder, doctors' responses to it will change—as will the responses of insurance companies and others involved with health-care delivery. Professional and lay organizations will also provide widespread support and information to those who suffer from headache. All of these factors should help those with headache to recognize that they are suffering from a genuine biological disorder, about which they need feel no remorse, guilt, or shame.

In this spirit, we hope that our book will be a useful aid to the many headache sufferers we have known, whose willingness to persist in the search for treatment continues to inspire our work.

(1)

THE PAIN IN YOUR HEAD

COPING WITH YOUR HEADACHES

As a chronic headache sufferer, you've probably heard a lot about why you suffer from headaches. You may even have come up with some theories of your own. The following statements—or statements like them—probably sound pretty familiar:

"Oh, come on, what's the big deal? It's just a little headache!"

"I don't believe you've got a headache at all. You're just trying to get out of going to visit my mother!"

"Why can't you just take an aspirin and forget about it."

"You must be upset about something. If you knew how to deal with your feelings, you wouldn't get headaches."

When you hear belittling statements like the ones above—even if you're the one telling them to yourself—you may feel angry, frustrated, despairing, embarrassed, guilty, or some combination of all of them. After all, you're the one who's experiencing the pain. You're the one who knows how bad it is. Why would you bring something so unpleasant on yourself?

You're also the one who knows that taking an aspirin just doesn't seem to help. Or if it does, you may be worried about how often you seem to need aspirin or some other headache medication. You may have noticed that your preferred medication or dosage seems to be less effective than usual, leaving you with apparently no protection at all against the pain of a headache. You're frightened, upset, in pain—you certainly don't want to hear that all you've got is some minor problem, or that you're somehow "making it all up."

Yet the idea that there are positive steps you can take to manage and prevent your headaches may come as an enormous relief. How wonderful if there really were something you could do to keep the pain away, or to drive it away once it comes. How wonderful to have confidence in your own ability to protect yourself from the tortures of a headache. For many people, the fear that a headache will come, or that it will somehow "last forever" is even greater than the pain of the headache itself. How wonderful to be free of all that, once and for all!

Well, this wonderful prospect is actually a reality. There are concrete steps that you can take to keep headaches away, and to reduce or eliminate your suffering when they do come. There are both prescription and off-the-shelf medications as well as medicine-free ways to manage your headaches; even, in some cases, to eliminate them or reduce them to minor nuisances rather than the painful recurring problems that they currently seem to be.

In order to take these steps, you will probably find it helpful to take responsibility for your headaches. That doesn't mean blaming yourself for them, feeling guilty about them, or deciding that you're somehow "bad" for having them in the first place. Indeed, such negative feelings will probably make your suffering even worse!

What will be helpful, however, is to understand that there is a complex relationship between your mind and your body. No one completely understands this relationship yet. Every day science is discovering new ways in which mind and body interact. What we do know is that emotions, brain chemistry, exercise patterns, muscle tone, and diet all seem to be involved in the experience we call a headache. And you can affect each one of these factors to reduce your headache pain.

YOU ARE NOT ALONE

In this chapter, we'll briefly describe the biology of your brain and explain the physical basis of pain. We provide this information because we believe that the more you know about how your body works, the more you'll be able to make satisfying and effective decisions about how to cope with your headaches. We'll also talk about the complex relationship between your mind and your body, and how this relationship determines your experience of a headache—and your ability to prevent and reduce headache pain. We'll talk about what you can expect from your doctor or other health care practitioner—and what you can't. And we'll make some suggestions for working with your physician.

First, however, we'd like to reassure you: You are not alone. The list of famous people who suffered from headaches is long, indeed. Karl Marx, Virginia Woolf, Miguel Cervantes, Lewis Carroll, Sigmund Freud, Frederic Chopin, Charles Darwin, Ulysses S. Grant, Thomas Jefferson, Peter Tchaikovsky, and George Bernard Shaw all suffered from headaches. So, reportedly, did Julius Caesar.

In our own time, some 90 percent of all people in the United States get at least some kind of headache some of the time, with 20 percent of the population going so far as to seek medical help for their headache pain. Some 50–70 million people a year complain of chronic pain in this country, and 40 million of them seek medical help.

Headaches are a profitable industry for some. In 1981, people in the United States spent about $500 million for off-the-shelf medication for headache pain. The total bill for lost work time, health care, and medication for this syndrome is about 6 to 8 billion dollars a year.

As you can see, headaches are a common syndrome. In this book, we'll show that they are often a misunderstood one. Contrary to popular opinion, there's quite a bit that you can do to reduce and prevent your headaches—sometimes without using medication.

A drug-free approach has some advantages over the use of medication, although it's not always possible to dispense with medication entirely. While medication may bring on occasional harmful side effects, a drugless approach usually encourages positive side effects, including weight loss, improved sleep, increased energy, and a general sense of well-being and calm. While medication may require larger and larger doses to maintain effectiveness, a drug-free approach continues to combat headaches as long as it is practiced. By making changes in your diet, your exercise patterns, and/or your ways of dealing with stress, you can substantially reduce and prevent your headache pain.

The first step in this process is understanding. Being able to imagine how your body works will help you increase your body awareness, as well as help you understand the impact of various treatments, both with drugs and without.

YOUR BRAIN AND YOUR BODY

Your body is controlled by two systems: the nervous system, which includes the brain, the spinal cord and its surrounding nerves—and the chemical elements that carry messages among these various entities; and the endocrine system, which includes the glands, and the hormones that help your glands communicate with one another. In addition, the nervous system and the endocrine system are also interrelated.

Both the nervous system and the endocrine system may be involved in your headaches. Pain, however, is a function of the nervous system.

The nervous system is set up to enable instant communication throughout the body. If you burn your finger, the awareness that you have done so is immediately processed by your brain. If your brain decides that you need to shy away from a hot fire, the impulse to draw back is immediately received by your hand.

WHERE IS HEADACHE PAIN LOCATED?
Interestingly, the brain itself can't feel pain. There are no pain-sensitive nerves inside the brain. If a surgeon were

cutting into the brain itself, an alert, awake patient would not experience pain.

The brain is well protected from outside dangers, as well. It's enclosed inside the cranium, or skull. Within the skull, it's cushioned by protective coverings called meninges, and it floats in a pool of cerebrospinal fluid that protects it further.

The skull, however, is covered with muscles, which are fed by blood vessels and served by nerves. The meninges are also sensitive to pain, as are the blood vessels right around the meninges.

Pain felt by muscles on the skull is known as *extracranial* pain—pain produced outside the cranium. In all likelihood, that's where your headache pain is located. *Intracranial* pain, or pain produced inside the cranium, is extremely rare. Usually, it's caused only by a brain tumor, blood clot, or blood vessel malformation, conditions found in less than 1 percent of headache sufferers. It's extremely rare that a headache would be the first sign of a brain tumor. Usually, any tumor large enough to cause pain (which would result from the tumor's pressure on the meninges or blood vessels) would first have caused dizziness, impaired vision, and other dramatic symptoms.

Your headache pain, then, has its physical source *outside* your brain, in the nerves leading to the blood vessels and muscles around your scalp, face, and neck. The eyes, ears, jaw, sinuses, and teeth are also sensitive to pain. And this pain may also feel like it's coming from inside your brain, even though it isn't.

Although your pain is stimulated by something happening to pain-sensitive nerves outside the brain, your brain is the real source of all your headache pain—and all your other pain as well. All sensory impulses are ultimately received by your brain—and that's where you perceive them as pain.

All physical sensations in the human body are a result of the "decisions" made by the brain about what to feel and how to interpret the feeling. Knowing how the brain works will help make this clear.

THE STRUCTURE OF THE BRAIN

The human brain is made up of billions of cells. Many of these cells have specialized functions. For example, some are sensory cells: they receive messages about sensory experiences (hot, cold, painful, soothing). Some are motor cells: they send messages about body movement (breathe, blink, move your hand, run). Other cells store memories, instruct glands to secrete hormones, and so on.

These specialized cells tend to be located in specific areas of the brain. Thus scientists can pinpoint the physical location within the brain that is responsible for sensory information.

The brain itself can't feel pain, as we've said. But the sensory cells in the brain interpret feelings of pain that occur elsewhere in the body. Thus, if the sensory portion of the brain were destroyed, you could burn your finger and feel no pain. In fact, there's even an operation that can be performed to remove the capacity to feel pain. As you can imagine, this is an extremely dangerous operation: without the ability to feel pain, you might severely damage a limb or vital organ without even being aware of it.

YOUR BRAIN AND YOUR SPINAL CORD

The brain is made up of two giant lobes, or hemispheres—the right hemisphere and the left hemisphere. These lobes rest on a stalk of tissue known as the brain stem. The brain stem is the "control center" of the body. It is the oldest part of the brain that controls the most primitive, basic aspects of the human body: staying conscious, keeping the heart beating, regulating blood pressure, and continuing to breathe. While all of these activities may be affected by our thoughts, they can also continue without us thinking about them.

On the back of the brain stem is a portion of the brain called the cerebellum. This part of the brain controls balance and coordination. Medications that treat pain often affect the cerebellum, which is why they include the side effects of dizziness and lack of coordination. Alcohol also affects the cerebellum; hence intoxication's staggering, clumsiness, and slurred speech.

The brain stem reaches down through an opening in the skull to the spinal cord, a bundle of nerves that carries messages to and from the brain throughout the body. The spinal cord is protected by the vertebrae, and is also covered by meninges and surrounded by cerebrospinal fluid.

The close connection between the brain and the spinal cord has led scientists to develop the *gate control* theory of pain. This hypothesis holds that there are two types of nerves that pass between spinal cord and brain. Nerve fibers, in large bundles, carry the sense of touch. Pain fibers, in smaller bundles, carry the sense of pain. If the touch fibers are overloaded, they can "close the gate" and block the messages of pain. That's why you may instinctively want to rub any part of the body that seems to hurt. The rubbing stimulates the touch nerve fibers, blocking the feeling from the pain fibers.

Pain nerve fibers are carrying messages from specialized cells in the skin and muscles that react to pain, pressure, temperature, and stretch. Every living organism, down to an amoeba, can feel pain. Apparently, specially shaped nerve endings designed to feel pain are a holdover from this more primitive stage of evolution, alongside our more complex sensory apparatus, which is capable of feeling more refined sensations. As you can see, the sensation of pain is extremely important to preserving life—such that even the one-celled amoeba must be able to feel pain.

Basically, you can picture your body as a network of nerve fibers, reaching into all parts of your body, connecting them with the spinal cord. In turn, your spinal cord is connected to your brain, through the brain stem, which in turn connects with the cerebellum and cerebral hemispheres (brain lobes).

Whenever a physical event occurs anywhere on your body—say, our old example of burning your finger—nerves instantly carry information about this event from the affected place, along the nerves, to your spinal cord, and finally, on up to your brain. Your brain receives this information in its sensory cells, and you experience the physical sensations that go with a burned finger.

INSIDE YOUR BRAIN

What happens when this information reaches your brain? It must be transmitted from one cell to the next, so that all of the brain's sensory cells can receive the information. This transmission is a fascinating process.

Each cell in the brain has extensions that reach out to neighboring cells. The extensions called axons are transmitters—they pass messages from one cell to the next. The extensions called dendrites are receivers—they receive the message. The space between a transmitter and a receiver is called a synapse.

How does a message cross a synapse? Scientists don't understand this process as well as we'd like. But we believe that various chemicals act as neurotransmitters. The neurotransmitter chemicals seem to play many functions. When the level of these chemicals changes within the brain, we may become more sensitive to pain. We may also have other brain-function disturbances, such as schizophrenia.

Some medications to combat headache pain may work by blocking this transmission of pain messages across synapses. Even though the cause of pain hasn't been removed, the pain is not experienced.

One of our most important neurotransmitters is called serotonin. Among its many other functions, serotonin seems to regulate our body's response to stress. It apparently has the ability to produce a state of relaxation. Serotonin is synthesized by our bodies from the amino acid (protein component) L-tryptophan, a substance found in green vegetables, fruits, dairy products, and turkey. (Because of toxic side effects, synthetically-produced tryptophan has been taken off the U.S. market.)

Other neurotransmitters that are activated when pain signals are transmitted include dopamine, norepinephrine, and acetylcholine.

Endorphins are another key chemical produced by our brains. Endorphins have a chemical structure remarkably like morphine. Both endorphins and morphine somehow affect the transmission of messages from one nerve to the next, in a way that somehow lessens pain. The body's natural ability to anesthetize itself explains why ballet dancers may sustain an injury that they don't even notice until after the show is over—when they may suddenly experience intense pain. Likewise, soldiers in battle or athletes on the field have been known to be unaware of their injuries for some time.

Apparently, laughing, regular aerobic exercise, and being in love all stimulate the body's endorphin production. So the more you practice any or all of those three activities, the more "immunity" you're building up to your headaches. On the other hand, depression may in part be biologically related to the body's underproduction of endorphins. Interestingly, many migraine people also suffer from depression. Raising the body's endorphin production may be of key importance for people with headaches.

The body's natural endorphin production may be impaired when you take medication to relieve pain. That's why most pain medication tends to be less effective after continued use, requiring you to take higher and higher doses in order to achieve the same effect. It's also part of why depression is sometimes associated with frequent intake of narcotic medication, even if the medication is effective in preventing or relieving headaches.

Referred Pain

Your body has twelve paired cranial nerves that carry information to and from your brain, as well as thirty paired spinal nerves that carry information to and from your spinal cord.

Because each nerve carries messages to and from many parts of the body, we sometimes experience the phenomenon known as *referred pain*. This means that, although the stimulation is taking place in one part of the body, the pain is felt elsewhere. Thus, when someone has a heart attack, they sometimes feel the pain in their arm instead.

Referred pain accounts for our frequent misperception of various headaches. Only one nerve, the fifth cranial nerve, carries messages to and from the face, eyes, forehead, sinuses, mouth, and meninges. Thus, when there is a strain on our jaw, we may feel pain behind an eye. When blood vessels are swelling in our temples, we may experience the pain as "inside our head," in the meninges.

This phenomenon also accounts for people's frequent perception that they have sinus headaches, that is, pain that radiates out from their sinuses. In fact, only about 10 percent of so-called "sinus headaches" actually refer to trouble with the sinuses. If your sinus headaches are not accompanied by such symptoms as a running nose, postnasal drip, and/or a fever, your headaches are probably not originating in your sinuses. However, you may experience them there, thanks to referred pain.

ISCHEMIC PAIN

There's one other type of pain that you should understand. It's called ischemic pain, and it's the pain that comes to a part of the body that experiences a lack of blood.

If you were to put a blood pressure cuff on your arm, so that your forearm was not receiving any blood, you would not experience any pain, even if you managed to stop circulation. However, if you tried to "work" with that arm, to move it or exercise it in any way, you would begin to feel pain.

Why? Apparently, exercising one's muscles produces metabolic waste products, which irritate the nerves and cause pain. When the blood circulates freely, it flushes out these waste products. Thus, if you took off the cuff and restored circulation, you would find that the pain would soon subside.

This process is important in understanding why our liver's activity may be involved with headache pain. The liver's role is to flush out toxins from the blood. A liver that is overworked by poor diet or too much alcohol cannot adequately cleanse toxins and waste products that may cause pain.

This process also helps explain why disturbances in blood circulation are related to headache pain. You can see that the more aerobic exercise you get, the more freely your blood will flow through your body, cleansing it of toxins that may produce pain.

WHAT IS PAIN?

As we have seen, pain is a complex biological interaction between your nerve endings and your brain. No matter what seems to "cause" pain—a slap, a wound, a headache—pain is not something "out there." It's something inside you.

When you receive an outside stimulus to pain, such as stubbing your toe on a step, the nerve endings in your foot are irritated. They are receiving the message that something traumatic has happened to your body, something that would probably not be good for your body to continue undergoing. This irritation in the nerve endings—pain—is your body's way of protecting itself, so that you take steps to stop the thing that is causing the pain.

What happens after the nerve endings are irritated? Nerve cells, or neurons, fire chemicals, or neurotransmitters, to carry the message they receive through other neurons along to your brain. Your brain must receive and interpret the message.

That's what we mean when we say that the pain is "inside" you. Stubbing your toe happened "outside" you—between your toe and the stair. But experiencing the feeling of the "stub" and interpreting it as unpleasant—that's the work of the brain, which takes place inside your head.

This is why people have all sorts of different reactions to outside physical stimuli. Some people are very sensitive to pain. Their brain interprets even the slightest outside stimulus as extremely dangerous, unpleasant, or intense. People who have been sick for a long time, for example, are often sensitized to even tiny pains in this way. Or you yourself may notice that when you have a headache, even the slightest noise or light strikes you as painful.

As you can see, the brain's interpretation of pain is an important part of our experience. Likewise, our reactions to an event can literally produce chemical changes in the brain that translate into painful sensations. Think about the last bad fight you had with a loved one. Don't you feel your stomach knotting, your jaw clenching, your back stiffening?

These physical sensations are just as real as any others— but their cause does not derive from a physical event, like stubbing your toe. Their cause is in your mind and your memory.

Many doctors now believe that people who suffer from headaches, particularly from migraines, are not classifiable by any particular personality type. The old idea that migraine or tension headache sufferers were more driven, more repressed, or more frantic than other people is not necessarily true.

What does seem to be true, though, is that people who suffer from headaches *translate* their stress into headaches, rather than into some other form. Because of the biochemical nature of their brains, experiencing the emotion of stress is one factor that can set off a physical chain reaction that produces the experience we know as a headache.

Of course, other factors may also trigger a headache. For some people, certain foods, alcohol, or dazzling lights might set off an attack. Women may be especially vulnerable to headaches just before, during, or just after their periods. It's also possible that some headaches have a kind of internal rhythm of their own, or have some other relation to body chemistry that we don't yet understand.

Some headaches may be a person's response to a stressful event or memory. There may be some other emotion, such as anger or guilt, that is being translated into the physical sensation of a headache. Or there may be some more physical cause, such as a poor posture, cigarette smoke, or alcohol.

Whatever the initial cause, what happens once the headache has been set off? Remember that the headache is literally happening "inside your head." That is, although the nerve endings that are being irritated are probably outside your head, on your scalp or along the back of your neck, the actual pain is being interpreted by your brain. Your response to this physical event can have a big impact on it.

That's why techniques like biofeedback, visualization, and relaxation exercises are effective for many people. All of these techniques are ways of harnessing your brain to interpret and react to the pain the way you want it to. These techniques work no matter what you think the cause of the pain is. They are good both for someone suffering from headaches and for, say, an athlete trying to increase his or her tolerance of the pain of running long distances. They work because they take advantage of the fact that your brain is always interpreting and deciding what pain is.

Pain and Suffering

We're used to equating pain with suffering, imagining that some objective physical event is acting upon our bodies. In order to separate the idea of pain from the idea of suffering, imagine for a moment some of the physical sensations which may cause you to "suffer," but which don't include physical pain.

Being in a place that is too hot or too cold is not literally "painful." But you may experience severe discomfort; you may even suffer. A strong, unpleasant odor does not "cause pain," but it may cause you to suffer if you cannot escape from it.

Now let's say that the odor that you find nauseating is the smell of someone cooking a spicy fish dish very early in the morning. Someone who regards this as his favorite dish might find the smell delicious. And you yourself might enjoy the odor later in the day—just not on an empty stomach! As you can see, your suffering is an individual experience, and one that is far more determined by your circumstances and state of mind than by the "objective" factor of the "bad smell."

The ultimate example of this concept is people who have had the operation known as a lobotomy. This operation severely interferes with the normal functioning of the brain. In some cases, people who have had lobotomies on account of experiencing severe pain say that after the lobotomy, they experience the same pain. However, it no longer bothers them.

Phantom Limb Pain

Another mystery of pain is phantom limb pain—the experience of some amputees that their lost limb "feels pain." This experience doesn't seem to be affected by medicating the remaining stump. Apparently, the brain retains memories of pain, memories that are so powerful that they may still be experienced, even when the original physical experience and even the original sensory apparatus (nerves in the lost limb) are long gone.

Just because this phantom limb pain is "all in someone's head," does that mean it isn't "real"? Of course not. The biochemical activity of the brain that corresponds to the experience of pain happens just the same, whether the stimulus for this activity is a physical event or a powerful memory. But for those of us who suffer from headaches, it's useful to know that a powerful memory or emotion may be the trigger for the biochemical event of pain.

PLACEBOS

In order to get the Food and Drug Administration's approval for a new headache remedy, drug companies must test the drug. Usually, they give the drug to one group of people in the experiment, and a *placebo* (a pill made of some inactive substance) to another group. Everyone hopes he or she is getting a "real" remedy—although they know the possibility exists that they are only getting a placebo. The idea is to see how many more people are "cured" by the real pill than by the placebo.

However, routinely, up to 40 percent of the group that gets the placebo experiences some headache relief. Think about that. Almost half of a randomly selected group of people feels some improvement in their headaches, just because someone told them that they were going to.

Some researchers theorize that placebos represent a form of self-hypnosis, in which the people taking the pill convince themselves that their pain will leave. Others believe the placebos are almost a form of hypnosis by the person giving the pill, since that person is usually an authority figure in whom the person receiving the pill has faith. Similarly, faith healing may be seen as a sign of the body's ability to heal itself, if only one's belief is strong enough.

HEALING YOURSELF

We certainly aren't providing these examples to convince you that you're somehow "making your headaches up." We believe that there is an objectively observable biochemical chain of events that produces the experience known as "headache pain." More information on what this chain of events is can be found in Chapter 2, as well as subsequent chapters.

Many different factors may trigger the chain of biochemical events that leads to a headache: something you eat, bright lights, weather, alcohol. Emotional experiences —feelings, memories, fears—may also trigger the process. On the other hand, many different factors may also modify this chain of events—precisely because it is so intimately bound up with your brain's decisions about how to interpret an event.

The fact that your brain interprets each event doesn't mean that you have total "control" over it. Most people's brains will interpret an event like, say, burning one's finger, as extremely painful (although we hear stories of people who are capable of walking on coals or sleeping on a bed of nails while feeling no pain, due to their long study of meditation and their intense awareness of the workings of their brain). However, if your brain did decide to interpret having your finger burned as a pleasant experience, you'd be in big trouble. Remember, even amoebas feel pain. Pain is your body's way of getting you to pay attention to something important, so that you'll take appropriate action.

Most of us in the West are used to thinking of the "mind" and the "body" as separate entities. For convenience, we'll talk about them that way, as well. But it's helpful to remember that in fact, from the point of view of the brain, there really is no difference. Every emotion, thought, or decision to act can be seen as a biochemical event within the brain. Whatever the original source of our thoughts and feelings, in order for us to think and feel them, they must have a physical presence, a biochemical event that takes place in the brain. That's why a physical event, like taking a tranquilizer or making love or going for a brisk run around the block, can help determine our emotions: because it has an effect on our biochemistry.

Likewise, emotions have a biochemical effect that affects our physical beings. Being nervous makes our stomach cramp up, our palms sweat, or our mouth dry out. Just thinking about someone we're attracted to can produce the same physical result as if that person were actually there.

Ironically, the biochemical result of experiencing constant pain is to make the body even more sensitive. This sensitivity expresses itself in both mind and body. Physically, the pain nerves are so irritated that they react more quickly to smaller stimuli. Emotionally, a person in constant or frequent pain tends to withdraw from others, in expectation that the pain will continue or get worse. Normally pleasant events are feared, because they might be an occasion for a terrible headache. This isolation increases the person's sense of depression and loss of control over his or her life. He or she is less likely to get the vigorous exercise that could increase the self-healing process of endorphin production. Such a person may also instinctively "brace" his or her body against the pain—causing muscle tension that increases the possibility of a headache. The pain becomes a downward spiral that is increasingly difficult to break.

What's the alternative? A person's willingness to play an active role in his or her own healing process. With the help of your doctor or health care practitioner, you can diagnose when you get headaches, what they feel like, and what seems to set them off. Working with a professional, or using the information in this book, you can discover the diet and exercise patterns that will help you resist the headache process. With a professional or by yourself, you can take a look at your emotional as well as your physical life, to see what may be causing you pain.

When you "put yourself in the driver's seat" in this way, you'll find that improvement in any area of your life will lead to gains in many other places as well. Eating better makes you feel better, so you have more energy to exercise. The exercise produces endorphins—chemicals naturally produced in the brain and similar in effect to morphine—which serve to improve your overall feeling of well-being. A positive attitude gives you the boost you needed to confront a difficult emotional situation, or to make some changes that you've always wished you could make. Each gain in one area provides a boost elsewhere, so that the downward spiral becomes an upward spiral.

Our approach to dealing with headaches is based on two principles:

One, you have a great deal of influence over the events that trigger the biochemistry of a headache in the first place. Diet, exercise, and the array of relaxation techniques mentioned above can eliminate some headache triggers from your life, and can vastly improve your body's ability to withstand the effects of a headache trigger.

Two, you have a great deal of influence over how you experience the biochemical events that make up a headache. Relaxation, creative visualization, biofeedback, and other techniques may help you react differently to headache pain. These differing reactions will themselves affect the biochemical processes going on in your head. This is an approach to *reducing pain.*

In other words, under some circumstances, you will react to drinking a glass of wine or to being yelled at by your boss by a biochemical chain of events that results in headache pain. But if you eliminate alcohol from your diet, or change your feelings about being yelled at, you may have eliminated the trigger that set the headache events in motion. Or, if you've made some changes in your diet, exercise pattern, or feelings about yourself and your life, your body may be able to resist its former impulse to translate alcohol or stress into the chain of events that produce a headache. This is an approach to *preventing pain.*

Our goal with this book is to give you all the information you need to decide how you want to respond to your headaches. Your biochemical makeup, the one that tends to produce headaches, is something you were born with. But your response to it is your responsibility—and your opportunity to begin to heal yourself.

WORKING WITH YOUR HEALTH CARE PROFESSIONAL

We've said a lot in this chapter about taking responsibility for your headaches. Does taking responsibility mean that you have to do it all alone?

Absolutely not. In fact, taking responsibility may make it possible for you to define the kind of help you need and then make sure that you get it. Whether you decide to see a medical doctor, a homeopath, a psychotherapist, a nutritionist, a masseur, or some combination of the above, you don't need to face your headaches alone.

WHEN YOU NEED TO SEE A DOCTOR

In some cases—very few—frequent, painful headaches may be the sign of some other, more serious condition. Although these conditions are rare, there are some 300 of them, including brain tumors, brain hemorrhage, meningitis, temporal arteritis, glaucoma, an infection, or a severe trauma, like a blow to the head, that has produced internal injuries. The treatment for these conditions is quite different from the response to "ordinary" headaches.

We recommend that you see a doctor to make sure that none of these conditions exist if you are experiencing any of the following symptoms:

- A headache associated with other neurological events, such as disturbances of vision or speech, numbness, weakness, or partial loss of feeling or control in a limb.
- Headaches that steadily increase in intensity, in frequency, or in the length of time they last.
- A sudden and extremely painful headache, like nothing you've ever felt before. This may be due to hemorrhaging or a ruptured aneurysm, and you should get yourself to an emergency room immediately.
- Headaches beginning after the age of fifty. They may be warning signs of some new disease. For example, new blood vessel problems in the heart or brain may cut down on the blood flow to the brain, which would

cause pain. An inflamed artery would also cause pain. Lung problems from long-term smoking or inhaling of polluted air might also cause headache pain; so might cancer, or mild increased pressure in the eyes. Arthritis of the neck vertebrae might cause pain that is in turn referred to the brain.

- Headaches associated with head injuries.
- Headaches that include other symptoms, such as fever, shortness of breath, or effects upon your eyes, ears, nose, or throat.
- Headaches associated with fever, stiff neck, nausea, and vomiting, which are symptoms that suggest meningitis.
- Headaches associated with memory loss and/or confusion.

THE MEDICAL HISTORY

Of course, you may also want to see a doctor or other health care practitioner even if the above checklist does not apply. If you do, what can you expect?

First, your doctor will probably take a medical history. Here are some of the areas you're likely to be asked about. (*Note:* if your doctor *isn't* looking at many or most of these factors, he or she may not be taking the right approach to your headaches—that is, one that acknowledges the interconnections of your body, your mind, and your feelings. We ourselves recommend such an approach, and would encourage you to seek a doctor who follows a similar one.)

Your Family   How did the family you grew up in handle difficulties? How did they handle anger? Is there any family history of migraine or "tension" headaches? How do you get along with your family of origin now?

Do you have a new family? Do you live with others or alone? Are you divorced? Do you have children with whom you live or whom you see regularly? Has there been a recent change in your living situation, such as a new roommate, a marriage, a new child, a child leaving home, or a divorce? How are you all getting along? Have there been any changes, either positive or negative, in your personal relationships?

Your Job What's your occupation? Do you have a supervisor? Do you supervise others? Do you work with others or alone? How are you getting along at work? Have there been any recent changes, either positive or negative, in your position, your coworkers, your salary, or your responsibilities? How do you like your job?

Your Medical History Are you allergic to any medications? How often do you drink, smoke, or take recreational drugs? (Since these factors can affect your headaches, it's important that you be absolutely honest with your health care practitioner about this.) Do you get regular exercise? What's your diet like? Are you concerned about your weight? Have you gained or lost weight recently, and do you have a pattern of gaining and losing weight?

Your Personal Life Do you have any hobbies? What do you do for fun? Are you frequently concerned about money? Do you wake up in the morning frequently feeling depressed, anxious, or with a feeling of dread? How would you describe your personality? Would you say that you are basically happy with your life, or that you'd like to make some changes? Is there something bothering you that you feel you can't control?

THE HEADACHE HISTORY

Next, your doctor will probably ask you for more information about your headaches. It will be useful for you to keep a headache diary, paying careful attention to the factors listed below, for about six to eight weeks. The headache diary may lead you to realize a few things even before you see your doctor!

YOUR HEADACHE DIARY

You may want to keep a headache diary, in which you note the thoughts, feelings, and events of each day, along with noting when you have headaches and what your experience of the headache is. (For a suggestion on what such a diary might look like, see the Appendix.)

We suggest buying either a large appointment book or a special notebook, and then reserving it for this purpose only. It may be helpful to arrange the book so that each pair of facing pages represents a "week at a glance," since many headaches follow a weekly pattern.

At the end of each day or the beginning of the next day, jot down what you ate, how you spent the morning, afternoon, and evening, any outstanding events, and how you felt for the three main parts of the day. You may find yourself wishing to write more, or you may only feel like making a few notes. Either way, stay as close as you can to writing about every day by the following morning, so that each day's mood stays separate.

On the days you get headaches, put your own headache symbol down in red, either an "H" or some other word or symbol that seems to express a headache to you. If thoughts or feelings come up as you mark this symbol down, record them, but don't ask yourself to think consciously about "why" you're getting headaches. Just record the events and feelings of each day, allowing yourself a fresh start every morning.

Then, after six or eight weeks, go back and notice when you got headaches. Perhaps you won't notice any patterns, but chances are, you will. These may be physical patterns —you get headaches whenever you sleep late, drink, or miss your morning coffee. Or they may be emotional patterns—headaches follow fights with your spouse (or times when your spouse made you mad and you *didn't* fight!), bad days at work, or good times with friends.

As the patterns become clear to you, you will be able to identify some of the kinds of changes you want to make. The relaxation techniques and others in this chapter may be helpful to you. With your increased awareness, you'll be able to choose the techniques that will be right for you.

What type of pain do you have? Is it throbbing or rather the sensation of a tight, squeezing band? Where does it seem to be located? Is it on one side of the head or both? Different headaches may be experienced differently; be sure you can describe each type of headache you're aware of to your doctor.

How intense is the pain? If you've kept a headache diary, it will be useful for you to rate your headache pain on a scale of one to three, in which one represents a mild headache, two a moderate to severe one, and three an incapacitating headache that prevents you from functioning. If you are seeing a doctor without the diary, give him or her some indication of how your headache pain varies or does not vary in intensity. Is it mild? Can it be incapacitating?

How long do your headaches last? Again, it will be useful to have kept a diary. If not, be as precise as possible as to the range of time your headaches usually last. Do they go on for one or two hours, all day, or constantly?

When did you get your first headache? Both the age and the circumstances of this headache would be helpful to your doctor.

Are your headaches associated with your period in any way? Many women get headaches only around the time of their period, or get especially severe headaches at that time. Menstrual migraines are a distinct syndrome, so begin to notice if there is a relationship between your headaches and the time of the month.

What happens the day before you get your headache? What happens just before you get your headache? The accumulation of this kind of information makes a headache diary useful. It enables you to "play detective," searching out the physical or emotional events that might trigger your headaches. If you aren't keeping a diary, think back to the last several headaches and ask yourself if they happened within a day or so after any of the following events: drinking alcohol, eating something sweet, missing a meal, having a disagreement with another person, taking on a new responsibility, successfully completing a task.

Many other events might trigger a headache, so allow your intuition to wander through the possibilities. Share your thinking with your health care practitioner.

How often do you usually get headaches? Has the frequency changed recently? If the latter is so, again, can you think of a change in diet, exercise, or emotional circumstances that preceded the change in headache patterns?

THE PHYSICAL EXAM

In all probability, your health care practitioner won't find it necessary to conduct a neurological examination, or to involve any of the more sophisticated tests we now have for monitoring brain function. We, however, believe that every headache patient deserves a complete history and neurologic examination performed by their health practitioner.

If so, you may be given a neurological exam. Your doctor may ask you some basic questions about recent events that happened, in order to test your short-term memory. You may be asked to interpret a proverb, such as "Don't bother locking the barn door after the horse has gone," in order to test your ability to think abstractly. You may be asked to perform mathematical calculations, in order to test your ability to compute.

If your doctor is giving you such a mental status examination, don't be concerned that he or she thinks your problem is "psychological." Rather, your doctor is making sure that all portions of your brain are working properly.

The doctor may also examine your cranial nerves (the twelve nerves that carry information to and from the area around the head and face); give you a motor examination to test your strength, reflexes, and coordination; or test your reaction to various sensory stimuli, such as being stroked with cotton, or pricked with a pin. Sensory exams may also test your sensitivity to vibration by placing a tuning fork at your wrist or ankle. The doctor may wriggle one of your fingers or toes into a certain position, out of your sight, and ask you to say whether it is pointing up or down; he or she may also ask you to identify by feel a letter or number "written" on your palm when your eyes are closed.

A doctor conducting these tests should make sure that you are fully aware of what is being done, and why. If it's not possible to give you this information while you are being tested, you should at least have a full explanation afterwards. You have a right to know what your doctor's concerns are—in other words, what he or she is testing for. You should also be able to ask any questions or express any concerns you have about your headaches or your treatment. Your doctor can't accomplish much without your trust—but he or she only deserves your trust if you sense that you are respected and acknowledged as an equal partner in your own treatment.

Sometimes a doctor will order further tests to check for

physical disorders. Blood tests and urine tests may be ordered to see if you are suffering from any medical problem that might be causing your headache. Your doctor may want to use x-rays to take a CAT (computerized axial tomography) scan in order to see whether you have any tumors, hemorrhaging, or blood vessel abnormalities, as well as to check the possibility of a previous skull injury or deformity. An x-ray of your neck may reveal arthritis, a fracture, or some other problem that could cause a headache.

While x-rays cause no immediate pain, they do expose you to a certain amount of radiation. They should never be ordered unless absolutely necessary, and they should never be ordered for a woman who is pregnant except in rare situations. If a woman has been sexually active without using contraception, she should consider herself potentially pregnant, and have an x-ray only during her period or the first five days after it. Of course, in an emergency, the value of an x-ray might outweigh the dangers.

Other medical procedures include electroencephalograms (EEGs), evoked potentials, facial thermography, MRI (magnetic resonance imaging) scans, cerebral arteriography, lumbar punctures, and Doppler ultrasound testing. Some of these tests are painful; others are quite expensive. Before performing any of them, your doctor should explain what the procedure involves and why it is necessary. You should have a good understanding of the costs and benefits involved, and be an active partner in the decision.

THE DOCTOR'S RESPONSIBILITY: A CHECKLIST

As you may already have experienced, some doctors can be dismissive or disrespectful of people with headaches. Far too many tend to prescribe too much pain medication, without encouraging their patients to explore drug-free methods of reducing or preventing headache pain. These same doctors are also likely to disregard their patent's complaints about side effects.

Some 70 percent of migraine sufferers are women, whom many doctors are especially prone to dismiss as "hysterical" or "just a hypochondriac." If you are a man or a woman who suffers from headaches, you know that your pain is very real. You have a right to be treated with respect, and to work actively with your doctor to find an effective solution to your problem. Here is our checklist of questions you may want to ask yourself about your health care practitioner. If you're not satisfied with the answers, you may want to find another person to treat your headaches.

- Are you treated with respect? Do you have a chance to explain your concerns both about your headaches and about your treatment?
- Does your practitioner explain fully the possible beneficial and side effects of any medication? Are you able to call him or her, either to discuss problems on the phone or to receive speedily another appointment to review problems in person? Has your doctor explained the difference between side effects that constitute an emergency versus side effects that warrant a phone call or quick appointment?
- Is your practitioner open to drug-free ways of dealing with headaches? Even if you are also receiving medication, are you being encouraged to examine your diet, exercise patterns, and psychological situation as well? Is your practitioner content to have you taking medication indefinitely, or is he or she committed to getting you off medication in the foreseeable future?

HOW TO USE THIS BOOK

Headache Relief doesn't offer any magic recipes or cure-alls. There may be some headaches that you cannot prevent, some headache pain that you cannot reduce.

On the other hand, you probably have a lot more resources at your disposal than you have guessed before this.

First, you have physical resources. Exercise has been found literally to alter the chemistry of your brain for a time, an alteration that has been extremely beneficial to many who suffer from headaches. Diet and vitamins obviously affect your body chemistry; the more you understand about them, the more you can develop the physical regimen that works for you. Certain techniques, like massage, acupressure, and facial and neck exercises, have been found very effective in reducing headaches in many cases.

Second, you have emotional resources. You can learn more about the emotional stresses that may trigger headaches, which is the first step toward managing those stresses in another way. You can learn about bringing your emotions in on the side of curing your headache ("I'll visualize a peaceful lake, and reward myself for trying to cope differently") rather than on the side of panic and anxiety ("All I can think about is how awful the pain is—what's wrong with me?"). And you can learn about some specific techniques—visualization, biofeedback, cognitive-behavior therapy—that may be helpful to you in headache management.

This book is your resource. You may want to read it straight through, noting what seems useful to you and ignoring what seems irrelevant. You may want to turn to the index or table of contents and read only the portions that interest you. Whatever you choose, remember that ultimately, this book is not the authority—you are. Whatever their initial cause, your headaches take place inside you. You are the one interpreting and experiencing the pain. You can be the one to prevent, reduce, and even cure it.

[2]

THE PHYSICAL BASIS
OF HEADACHES

THE WAY YOUR HEAD IS MADE

As we explained in Chapter 1, the brain itself doesn't feel any pain. Headache pain has its source in the nerves located in the muscles and blood vessels of your face, neck, and scalp, and in the nerves running between the back of the brain (the brain stem) and the brain's blood vessels. If you can understand the different parts of your head, you can visualize more clearly what's happening when you get a headache. As we'll see in Chapters 4 and 5, being aware of what's happening within your body is one step toward being able to affect it.

MAJOR ARTERIES

One of the major arteries outside your skull is called the *temporal artery*. It comes up from the neck, runs below and in front of your ears, and forward to your upper temple, where it divides and runs over your forehead.

The other major artery that serves the muscles of your scalp is the *occipital artery*. This vessel also runs up from the neck, up the back of your head. It goes beneath and behind the ears on each side. Then it divides from each side and runs across the lower back of the skull.

MAJOR MUSCLES

The muscles on your head help you move different parts of your face, your jaw, and your scalp. These muscles overlap the muscles of the neck and are connected to the muscles of your shoulders. Your spinal column—a column of vertebrae, or backbones, stacked like building blocks, is held in place by the *paraspinal muscles*. These muscles go up to the base of the skull, where they overlap other muscles going down the neck and into the shoulders. Together, they control the movements of your head, neck, and shoulders.

On the side of your head are the *temporalis muscles,* which cover the area in front of and above your ear, along the side of your skull (temples). These muscles are attached to your lower jaw. If you put a finger between the top of your ear and the corner of your eyebrow and then clench your teeth, you'll feel the movement of this muscle. Astute watchers of body language always look to the temporalis muscle; tightness there is one of the surest indicators of hidden tension.

The *frontalis muscle* covers the front of your head and forehead, like a cap. This is the muscle that you use to raise your eyebrows or move your scalp forward. It's also a muscle in which you may experience headache pain.

The many small muscles around the eye—which enable you to blink, squint, and open your eyes wider—interact with the frontalis muscle. Thus tension in one area may spread to the other.

On the back of your head is the *occipitalis muscle*. This muscle covers the lower back portion of your skull, a portion of your scalp that doesn't move. However, this muscle does surround the occipital artery. If the occipitalis muscle contracts, the occipital artery feels the pressure. As we shall see, this relationship also has consequences for headache pain.

The rear base of your skull is connected to the upper vertebrae (backbones) of your neck. The neck muscles around these vertebrae allow you to move your head. These muscles overlap the shoulder muscles as well.

One of the major muscles involved with headache pain

is the *trapezius*, or *shoulder muscle.* This triangular muscle covers your shoulder blades. It continues on up to your skull, extending all the way up to the small knobs behind your ears (mastoids).

The trapezius is also involved with your body language. One of the most common human reactions to a difficult situation is to hunch the shoulders. This seems to be an instinctive reaction that has its ancestry in animal behavior. Turtles, for example, are able to withdraw their heads and necks into their shells. Some apes, when threatened, seem to raise their shoulders and try to withdraw their heads down between them.

This bracing motion requires tensing the trapezius. Shrugging or bracing your shoulders contracts the trapezius, which may pull on the pain sensors in the muscle tissue. This pulling in turn may put pressure on the occipital artery that runs up the back of your skull.

Later in this chapter we'll look at the various types of headaches and their physical bases. Knowing the structure of the blood vessels and muscles on your head will make it easier to understand what happens when you have a headache.

HEADACHES CAUSED BY BRAIN TUMORS

Many people's first reaction to severe or chronic headaches is to worry that something even more serious is the matter. Sometimes, there is another problem at the root of the headache pain: about 10 percent of those who seek help for headaches have some organic disorder of which the headache is a symptom. However, less than 1 percent of those seeking help for headaches have brain tumors.

As we said in Chapter 1, a headache is very rarely the first or only sign of a brain tumor. Usually it's accompanied or preceded by vomiting, personality changes, noticeable changes in mental functioning—including difficulty in concentrating, drowsiness, seizures, or fainting. The headache pain feels like a tight band squeezing the head, but there is also a persistent pain that seems to be concentrated in one area and that seems to build. The pain of a brain tumor headache may wake a person from sleep, and the pain increases, whenever the person coughs, strains, or suddenly moves the head.

The pain of a brain tumor comes from the tumor pressing against the meninges, or brain covering, within the skull, or against the major arteries or sinuses. Because the brain can feel no pain, the tumor must grow quite a bit before it can reach a portion of the body that does feel pain. Before that has happened, the tumor's pressure is likely to produce the symptoms described above, which are actually disturbances in brain functioning. That's why a headache is usually one of the last signs of a brain tumor.

Patients with brain tumor exhibit a variety of symptoms. We treated a forty-six-year-old man with a long-standing history of cluster headaches that had been kept under good control for many years. He began to notice some difficulty with his driving: he tended to drive his eighteen-wheel rig off to the right side of the road and often ended up on the shoulder. At times, he even had trouble remembering how to get back to the truck yard.

He began to have moderately severe, steady, generalized headaches which gradually became worse and worse. He suffered from nonthrobbing pain associated with nausea and vomiting and was slightly unsteady on his feet.

We performed a neurological exam and discovered weakness on his right side as well as an inability to see objects from his right side. Emergency CAT scans of the brain and lungs showed a tumor in the left side of his brain as well as cancer of the lung which had spread to the brain. These had been causing his worrisome symptoms.

After underging surgery to remove the lung and brain tumors, he has improved significantly and has been able to resume his job.

OTHER ORGANIC CAUSES OF HEADACHES

An "organic cause" for a headache is some other physical condition besides the headache syndrome itself, a condition of which the headache is just a symptom. As we said, organic causes account for about 10 percent of the headaches of people who seek help.

Conditions that may cause headaches include hemorrhaging into the layers of the meninges (brain covering) or into the brain itself, ruptured aneurysms, meningitis, and temporal arteritis. For a list of the severe symptoms that indicate the possible presence of these conditions, see page 36 in Chapter 1.

Another condition that may cause headache is a problem with the muscles or joints of one's jaws. If chewing hurts, if your jaw opens abnormally, or if you tend to grind or clench your teeth, especially at night, you may have a dental or jaw problem. If in addition to these symptoms you have headache, earache, or face pain, the pain in the jaws or joints may be referred up to these other areas, so that you experience it as a headache.

Finally, eye problems may be experienced as a headache. Glaucoma is an eye disease caused by increased pressure in the eyeball. As glaucoma develops, the eye gradually becomes covered with a white film, and a person frequently experiences acute throbbing pain around, or behind, the eye and in the forehead. The person may also see halos or rings around lights, or have red eyes. Again, this eye pain is often referred to other areas of the head, so that it feels like a headache.

If you have any of these symptoms, or if your headaches are so persistent or severe as to interfere with your work or personal life, you should certainly see a doctor in order to be sure that they don't represent a more serious condition.

MUSCLE CONTRACTION OR "TENSION" HEADACHES

WHAT IS A MUSCLE CONTRACTION HEADACHE?

Some 75 to 80 percent of the headaches that people get fall into this category. And some 90 percent of the population gets this type of "tension" headache from time to time.

Although this type of headache may seem familiar, there are actually two types of muscle contraction headaches.

Acute headaches are temporary, specific responses to particular events. Many people get these headaches after a stressful time; this type of headache is usually responsive to a mild over-the-counter drug, a brief nap, or a short period of relaxation.

Chronic headaches, on the other hand, are frequent: at least twice a week, and extending up to seven days a week. Those who suffer from chronic muscle contraction headaches often wake up with a headache, or develop one early in the day.

Unlike classical migraines, muscle contraction headaches bring no warnings or "auras." They are usually not accompanied by vomiting and other symptoms. Nor is their pain disabling. In fact, people with chronic muscle contraction headaches are able to continue with their normal activities while the headache continues.

The pain in a muscle contraction headache is usually felt in the forehead and the back of the head and neck. The sensation is like having the head held in a vise. Although you have various perceptions of where such headaches begin, they actually begin at the back of the head most of the time. Then they radiate forward, reaching both sides of the head, although perhaps not with equal intensity. They may come up as far as the temples, or up to the area just behind the eyes, so that the whole head is "covered" by them.

Along with the head pain, people with these headaches frequently experience sore shoulders, and possibly a sore neck as well. Sometimes they can feel "knots"—tightly contracted muscles in the head, neck, or back.

There are many different patterns for muscle contraction headaches, but usually they occur during stressful times.

A frequent pattern for muscle contraction headache people is that they will work intensely for days at a time, until they have completed a week's duties. The work may be of the type where people are constantly trying to "beat the clock," to get a large amount of work done in a fixed

THE PHYSICAL BASIS OF HEADACHES / 51

amount of time, whether such work is inside or outside the home. Then, on their first day off, they will awaken with a headache. However, it's rare for such headaches actually to disturb a person's sleep.

It's also common for people to get muscle contraction headaches after staying in the same position—sitting, reading, typing, or driving—for a long time. Some people get these headaches from playing cards, from writing, or from working long hours at a desk.

Muscle contraction headaches can last for days without relief—except while the person is asleep. Relaxing seems to help these headaches, although frequently people with these headaches would prefer to be active. An occasional off-the-shelf analgesic can be helpful.

People with chronic muscle contraction headaches may be taking analgesics—aspirin, acetaminophen (Tylenol), ibuprofen (Advil), or some other headache medication—sometimes several doses a day. Usually, these pills have long since ceased to be effective. (For more on pain relievers of this kind, see Chapter 3.) However, chronic headaches may be eased by heat or cold applied to the back of the neck. Massaging the neck is also helpful. (For more on physical, drugless treatments of these headaches, see Chapter 6.)

Muscle contraction headaches usually begin in adult life. However, some 10 to 20 percent of people with this type of headache started getting them as children or teenagers. Men and women seem to get this type of headache about equally.

WHAT CAUSES MUSCLE CONTRACTION HEADACHES?

For many years, this category of headache was used as a kind of wastebasket. Any headache that didn't seem to fit other diagnoses was just tossed into this category. Likewise, as the name "tension headache" suggests, these headaches were largely attributed to emotional causes. The theory was that people who suffered from them were simply tense or repressed people whose bottled-up emotions caused them to contract their muscles, which somehow led to headache pain.

Now we think differently about so-called tension headaches. The very word tension is misleading, suggesting that tension is the root cause of the pain. In fact, we now believe that tension headaches are a by-product of a central nervous system disorder, probably the same disorder that also leads to migraines. Migraines and muscle contraction headaches are probably on a continuum, various aspects of the same disorder.

What is this disorder? We don't really know yet. We suspect that it involves the suppression of a major system within the brain, the *serotonergic* system, which controls sleep, the sensation of dull pain, emotions, and the sense of well-being. That may be partly why chronic muscle contraction headaches are often associated with depression and sleep disturbance, which may also involve the dysfunction of this system.

Whatever this disorder is, it seems be rooted in a biological predisposition that leads some people to translate various physical and emotional stresses into migraine headaches, and other people to translate these stresses into muscle contraction headaches. Sometimes, especially after many years, people with one type of headache develop the other (see the section on "Mixed Headaches," below), which is further evidence that the two types of headache are on a continuum, sharing a common source in the central nervous system.

Contracting one's muscles when facing danger seems to be an instinctive human reaction, along with pupils dilating, the heart muscle contracting more quickly, and the muscles in some blood vessels loosening to allow more blood to pass through. The muscles that contract are acting out a remnant of the body's "splinting" behavior, whereby muscles will contract tightly around a broken bone or other injured place to prevent further injury.

This emergency reaction takes place whether the danger we face is physical or emotional. That is, the body mobilizes for a physical threat even if the "danger" is having an argument with a loved one—or the memory of having the argument.

We don't know exactly why contracting muscles cause

pain, although we know this has something to do with the reduced blood supply to the area, which is failing to clean out metabolic wastes that build up, and that the blood-stream normally washes away. We do know that the pain of contracting one's muscles may be triggered by only two minutes of contraction, and that the pain may appear or continue long after the muscles are relaxed. That's why people can sometimes get headaches the day after the stressful events have ended.

In addition to a general tightening up of muscles, muscle contraction headaches seem to involve an instinctive hunching of the shoulders and drawing back of the head, much as a turtle pulls its head into its shell when threatened. This image of looking for a place to hide is a powerful one for many people with muscle contraction headaches.

Think of how tense or relaxed the muscles around your face, head, neck, and shoulders are. Look in the mirror, or do a body awareness check, working your way up from the bottom of your spine. Is there any pain or tightness in your lower back? Are your shoulders hunched? What happens when you try consciously to relax them or let them drop— do they tighten up in protest at the unfamiliar position, or creep up again into their usual protective position? How does the back of your neck feel—loose? tight? knotted?

What about your facial expression? Is it usually a frown? A serious look? A fixed smile? A look of anger? Do you frequently find yourself clenching your jaw, or grinding your teeth?

Running this physical check on yourself several times a day, particularly during times when you've got a lot to do, might help you understand how you are translating possible feelings of anger or worry into muscle contraction. Often, people with muscle contraction headaches aren't aware either that they are feeling angry or worried, or that their muscles are clenched. Becoming aware of both the feelings and the physical response is the first step to changing the headache pattern.

Another common pattern among people with muscle contraction headaches is to wake up in the morning with a headache. Possibly, this is a result of the uninhibited hours of sleep, when distressful feelings that have been ignored throughout the day finally come to the surface. Your body reacts to these feelings by contracting its muscles protectively, and you awake with a feeling of depression and a headache. Along with the image of a turtle wanting to pull its head into its shell, we might suggest the image of a bottle of difficult feelings. The aching head is the cork being pulled down into the bottle, trying literally to keep the lid on.

None of this means that you have more angry or worried feelings than other people, or that you have greater difficulty dealing with these feelings. It only means that your way of dealing with them, for whatever physical or psychological reason, is to translate them into muscle tension, which in your body is likely to lead to headaches. It may also mean that, in order to reduce or prevent your headaches, you will need to find a new way of coping with these feelings, so that muscle contraction and consequent headache pain does not result. (For more about the psychological bases of headaches, and some possible responses, see Chapter 5.)

PHYSICAL SOURCES OF MUSCLE CONTRACTION HEADACHES

It's also possible that your muscle contraction headaches are coming from a more physical source, such as arthritis, poor posture, or holding one position for a long period of time.

Arthritis is an inflammation of the joints. There are many types of arthritis. Rheumatoid arthritis is the most serious and the least common type, involving a rapid degeneration of the joints and the bones around them. Osteoarthritis is the most common type, which sooner or later affects nearly everyone. It comes from years of stress on a joint, which sooner or later causes it to become inflamed.

If joints in the neck develop arthritis, the muscles around them may instinctively be contracting in order to "splint" the pain. Or they may simply be braced against the pain—even though, paradoxically, this makes the pain worse.

If arthritis has led to the degeneration of a bone or spinal disc (the cartilage that acts as a cushion between each vertebra), this degenerating matter may press on a nerve that extends from the spinal cord. The nerve then becomes irritated and inflamed, a condition known as having a pinched nerve.

Because a pinched nerve is not fully functioning, this may lead to pain, tingling, numbness, or weakness in the area that the nerve serves. A pinched nerve in the neck or the lower back may refer pain down the entire arm or leg. A pinched upper cervical nerve may refer pain up into the head.

Any neck abnormalities are also possible orgins of a muscle contraction headache. Whiplash, a spinal tumor, or congenital (present from birth) deformities may put pressure on a nerve, causing pain and the consequent muscle contraction response to it. If you have a neck problem, it seems that any emotional stress is also more likely to trigger a muscle contraction headache, possibly because even a slight muscle contraction response to an emotional trigger sets up the vicious cycle of pressing on a nerve, and in turn causing greater contraction from the neck muscles.

If you have had an injury to your occipital nerve, from whiplash or a fall or blow at the back of the head, you will feel pain and tenderness from the base of your skull that radiates to the top of your head, or to your eyes. In this case the muscles around that nerve will tighten up protectively, which may also cause headache pain. Treatment for such a condition is unfortunately limited, since the nerve can't be "repaired" and must heal on its own.

MIGRAINE

Although the more extreme forms of migraine are well-known as "sick headaches," many people suffer from milder forms of migraine or migraine variants at various times in their lives. Technically, a migraine is defined as a headache that affects one side of the head. Usually it's accompanied by gastrointestinal disturbances, such as vomiting. Sometimes it's preceded by visual disturbances, known as the "aura." Most people who suffer from migraines have a family history of the condition. Migraineurs (people with migraine) often get headaches at certain times, such as on weekends, or around the time of menstruation.

Because the medical diagnoses of migraine can vary so much, it's hard to come up with precise statistics on how prevalent they are. Basically, though, we expect that some 8 to 10 percent of all men and 18 to 20 percent of all women have experienced a migraine at some point in their lives, for a total of 50 million people in the United States. Some 75 percent of all migraineurs are female, particularly in the hormonally active years between adolescence and menopause.

Migraine can begin at any time of one's life, although most people who are going to get migraines have gotten them by adolescence. Some studies have shown the following breakdown of migraine onsets: Twenty-five to 33 percent of all migraineurs have gotten their first headache by age ten; 56 percent by age thirteen; 75 percent by age thirty; and 90 percent by age forty.

As we've said, most migraineurs are women, and their migraines most frequently begin with the onset of their first period. On the other hand, of the 10 percent of migraineurs who get migraines after age forty, many are women who get their first headaches around the time of menopause.

Sometimes migraines disappear, or go into remission, for several years, only to reappear in the same or a different pattern. It's also possible for a person's migraine pattern to change as the headaches continue, so that headaches vary in frequency, in intensity, or in the kind of events that bring them on. This variation can of course be affected by treatment, but it appears to take place spontaneously as well.

SYMPTOMS OF A MIGRAINE

How do you know if your headaches are migraines? Final diagnosis may have to be made by a health care practitioner, but see if the following description fits:

A migraine headache may begin with seeing brightly

colored, blinking lines. This visual aura may also include flashes of lights, hallucinations, seeing only half of objects, or seeing spots of different shapes and colors. Before the headache, the migraineur may feel sensitive to bright light, especially to sunlight.

Then, the headache comes on swiftly, within ten to thirty minutes after this preceding aura. However, many migraineurs have no aura, are not aware of warning signs, or experience their warning symptoms (premonitory signs) for up to several days before the attack.

The headache, when it comes, lasts from eight to seventy-two hours. It may come during sleep, awaking the migraineur with its pain. It may come on around the menstrual cycle, or during the week before. Frequently, migraineurs get headaches when they've missed a meal, or gone for six hours without eating. Another common pattern is for a person to get a migraine right after a long period of stress, say on a weekend or a vacation. The migraine comes not during the stress, but during the "letdown" period afterwards.

Migraine may be experienced as dull, aching pain, or as severe, disabling pain. It usually begins in the temple or the eye. The pain may feel as though it's spread down to the neck, or sometimes, to the arm.

Generally, migraine pain is felt as intense and throbbing. Exposure to light, noise, or movement seem to make it worse. So does bending over. Sometimes migraineurs feel worse when they are sitting or standing, and seek a dark, quiet place to lie down. Occasionally a migraineur will feel the pain more intensely while lying down. Nausea and vomiting frequently accompany the pain, as does sensitivity to light and sound, dizziness, diarrhea, increased urination, and a feeling of not wanting to eat. For some, nausea and vomiting may be more debilitating than the pain.

A migraineur may feel cold while he or she is having the headache, particularly in the hands and feet. If so, he or she probably had a "hot head" during the period just before the headache began. These changes are partly caused by changes in circulation, but are also probably related to disturbances of the hypothalamus, the body's "thermostat."

Some migraineurs experience more pronounced symptoms. In severe cases, the migraineur will feel a tingling or numb sensation in the lips, tongue, or face, or in the fingers on the side where the pain is felt. There may be weakness on one side of the body or double vision.

A migraineur may also experience difficulty speaking or thinking. He or she may have a mild form of aphasia, in which the person is aware of what he or she wants to say, but is also aware that the words to express it aren't coming out correctly. In the most severe cases, a migraineur will experience bouts of amnesia during the headache. The migraineur's coordination is sometimes affected as well.

Occasionally, the pain seems to vary while the headache lasts. The pain may switch from one side of the head to the other, or it may seem to take over the entire head. Over the course of a lifetime, the migraine pattern may also change.

After the headache is over, the migraineur may feel a surge of energy and feel quite hungry. On the other hand, he or she may feel drained and washed out for days.

Although there tends to be a family history of migraine, it's often difficult to tell whether one's parents were in fact migraineurs. Their headaches may have stopped or decreased in frequency by the time their children were old enough to be aware of them. They may have mistakenly attributed the headaches to a sinus problem, or simply thought of them as sick headaches without labeling them as migraine.

Children with migraine may first have frequent and unexplained episodes of nausea, vomiting, or abdominal pain. If these children later develop a migraine pattern as teenagers or adults, their parents may not connect the two problems. (For more on children and migraines, see Chapter 10.)

What Causes a Migraine?

Migraines are in the category of headaches known as *vascular* headaches because they involve difficulties with the blood vessels in the face, head, and neck. Basically, these blood vessels are sometimes unnaturally narrowed, and other times abnormally widened.

Scientists have advanced various theories about the chain of events that represent a migraine, and about what sets off that chain. We know that vasoconstriction—the narrowing of blood vessels in the brain or in the vessels carrying blood to the brain—corresponds to the aura stage of the migraine. At this point, the brain is not getting enough blood, due to the constricted vessels. Lack of blood to the sensory portions of the brain seems to be the reason for hallucinations, visual disturbances, tingling and numbness, and other aspects of the aura.

Headache pain may involve inflammation of tissue around the blood vessels. If the blood vessels are unnaturally constricted, there will be an accumulation of chemical irritants within the vessels, since a normal flow of blood is not pulsing through to wash these irritants away. In fact, an excess of neurokinin, a substance similar to a material found in wasp venom, has been found in migraineurs during this stage.

The vasoconstriction seems to set off the opposite reaction: vasodilation (the widening of blood vessels on the surface of the brain and in the scalp). This corresponds to the throbbing, painful stage of migraine, in which it seems as though the head might burst from an excess of blood. In fact, part of the pain comes from the pressure on nerves in the blood vessels being stretched beyond their capacity as the vessels dilate to an unnatural width.

What sets off this process of constriction and dilation? Here again, scientists have advanced many theories. One hypothesis relates migraine to hypoglycemia, or a tendency to low blood sugar. For more detail on this theory, see pages 191–97 in Chapter 7.

A theory we find more convincing points to changes in the level of serotonin circulating within the brain, with the level especially high before migraines and unusually low during migraine. The effect of other vasoactive substances —substances that have an effect on the blood vessels' constriction or dilation—is also important.

Another theory, which doesn't necessarily contradict the others, focuses on the hypothalamus. This part of the brain is located behind the eyes and above the pituitary gland. The hypothalamus gets information from the part of the brain that experiences emotions, or the limbic centers. It transmits information to the pituitary, which regulates hormonal changes.

Through its influence on the pituitary and other glands, the hypothalamus controls body cycles, such as when one is hungry, when one sleeps and wakes, the timing of menstrual cycles, and other hormonal secretions. It also communicates with the brain stem, in which the body's pain-fighting system is located. Scientists believe that the brain stem has a system for modifying the body's ability to perceive incoming stimuli as painful. Thus our experience of pain is determined by the interaction between this pain-fighting system (which keeps us from feeling extreme pain at every bump and bruise) and the body's pain sensors (which keep us from easily tolerating the sensory experience of breaking a bone or being wounded).

In some way that we don't yet fully understand, the brain's neurotransmitters are involved in this complex perception of pain. As we discussed in Chapter 1, neurotransmitters are the chemicals that enable messages to be transmitted from one nerve cell to another within the brain. Neurotransmitters involved in the perception of pain include endorphins (the body's natural anesthetic), noradrenaline, and serotonin. Problems with the production and behavior of these neurotransmitters may lead to headaches.

It seems that the serotonin level in a migraineur's brain falls just before the migraine comes on. This corresponds to a drop in mood, like depression. Migraineurs often have a family history of depression, as well as a family history of migraine, again suggesting a biological connection.

Serotonin has the effect of constricting blood vessels. The relationship between serotonin and the conditions under which it comes into play is a complicated one that we are only beginning to understand.

We do know that serotonin is a nitrogen-containing substance called an amine. All of the amines—noradrenaline, histamine, and others—affect the blood vessels, sleep patterns, and a person's mood. It seems that a low level of amines may be associated with depression, while higher levels may be associated with mania, but again, this relationship is complicated. Migraineurs often find that food high in certain amines sets off a headache, along with the period of depression that precedes it. (For more on the relationship between amines and migraine, see Chapter 7.)

It's possible that the levels of amines may not be the issue at all. In laboratory studies, the blood vessels of migraineurs showed a greater sensitivity to serotonin than did the vessels of people without headaches. Likewise, migraineurs seemed to react more extremely to tyramine, a substance found in many foods, and to adrenaline, which is one of the substances known as the catecholamines. (For more on how these substances affect a migraineur and set off a headache, see Chapter 7.)

This hypersensitivity has led scientists to hypothesize that migraineurs may have a more "naked" sensory system than other people. In other words, sensations and experiences of the outside world seem to affect a migraineur's body chemistry more intensely and directly, as though the migraineur had no defenses against this stimulation.

Another substance involved in the brain's chemistry is a lipid (fat) called prostaglandin. One type of prostaglandin (PGE) stimulates blood vessels to expand, and seems to be set off by the constriction process that precedes a migraine. (For more on prostaglandins, see Chapter 7.) When people who had never had migraines were injected with this type of prostaglandin, they quickly developed symptoms that resembled the experience of a migraine headache.

This leads us to consider the hypothesis that migraineurs may have an extraordinary sensitivity to the amines, which leads their body to overproduce prostaglandins. It's the high level of prostaglandins, which is not normally found in nonmigraineurs, that may lead some people to have a migraine. This is not, however, the principal cause of a migraine, only one factor in some people's tendency to this type of headache.

Some scientists hypothesize that these body reactions

—which are closely related to the overproduction of adrenaline—are the primitive means by which the body responds to an emergency. Unfortunately, the "protection" which leads to a headache—is worse than any threat!

THE TWO MAIN TYPES OF MIGRAINES

CLASSICAL MIGRAINE

About 10 to 15 percent of all migraineurs get what are known as "classical" migraines or migraines with aura. These are easily the most dramatic form of migraine, because of the pronounced nature of the aura that precedes the headache.

The aura lasts some ten to thirty minutes before the actual beginning of the headache. It includes various types of sensory disturbances. Visual disturbances include: flashbulb-like blind spots in one or both eyes, sparkling areas in various colors, unusually shaped spots in either black and white or color, partial blindness in half of each eye, an irregular blind spot before the eyes (known as a *scotoma*), and tunnel vision (the inability to see to the sides). Some patients see wavy lines moving across their vision. A common aura is a crescent-shaped area composed of zigzag lines that blink lighter and darker, or shimmer, as they move slowly across the visual field.

Sometimes migraineurs think they have a period of clumsiness or a lack of understanding before their headaches, but this may simply be due to their inability to see properly.

A migraineur's aura may also include distortions in body image (seeing oneself as larger or smaller than is true), as well as other sensory disturbances in perceptions of shape, hearing, taste, smell, and touch. Lewis Carroll, the author of *Alice in Wonderland*, suffered from severe migraines. Possibly the distortions experienced by Alice were based on his own headache and aura experiences.

Other symptoms of the classical migraine may include numbness or tingling in various parts of the body; a sense of coldness, especially in the hands and feet; fever; fatigue; drowsiness; irritability; sweating; swelling in some part of the body (known as *edema*); abdominal pain; a feeling that the skin is too sensitive to be touched; confusion; slurring of one's speech; or aphasia (inability to find the right words, while being aware that one is unable). Sometimes classic migraineurs also need to urinate more often, or get diarrhea.

After the aura comes the headache phase, the period of actual pain. Frequently, the pain begins as mild, then gets worse. It's usually felt first in one side of the head, usually in the temple or behind the eye, though it may spread to both sides. The pain may be experienced in the head, as well as in the forehead, ear, jaw, back of the head (occiput), or all over. A person in the throes of migraine may feel that certain parts of the head are quite tender, especially the temple or neck.

Often classical migraineurs experience pain in their shoulders and backs. This is very likely the result of tightly contracted muscles in these areas: since moving the head seems to make the pain worse, the body is probably braced, trying to keep the head still. Thus the migraine headache is compounded by a muscle contraction headache as well. The duration of the pain in classical migraine is four to twelve hours.

After the migraine passes, the migraineur may have sore muscles. He or she may also feel exhausted or mentally "cloudy," as though still recovering from an intense experience.

The fact that people who frequently get classical migraines are also more likely to suffer from heart attack and stroke has led scientists to look at the blood circulation for clues to the migraine's cause. One theory is that platelets— the element in the blood that helps clotting—are abnormally sticky in migraineurs. Thus migraineurs are more likely than others to have their blood clot too easily. Aspirin seems to decrease the stickiness of platelets, which is why some studies have found it to help prevent heart attacks and stroke. However, these studies have also been challenged by various researchers, who have also pointed out some dangers of taking aspirin. (For more on aspirin and other pain relievers, see Chapter 3.)

Another factor is that blood platelets seem to carry neurotransmitters (our old friend, serotonin), which affect the size of blood vessels and the rate of clotting. Possibly, neurotransmitters on sticky blood platelets trigger the constriction of some blood vessels, producing the aura phase of migraine. Then, in reaction, the large blood vessels outside the skull dilate, stretching the nerve endings along the vessel walls, causing the headache pain.

COMMON MIGRAINE

Most people who suffer from migraine get so-called common migraine headaches, or migraine without aura, wherein a lack of distinct symptoms may lead to misdiagnoses. Although common migraines aren't preceded by a dramatic aura, there may indeed be warning signs that come hours or even days before an attack: a feeling of mental "cloudiness," weight gain, food cravings (especially for chocolate or sugar), fatigue, or extreme irritability. Some people also get swelling (edema) in some body part, or have an increased tendency to urinate, before the onset of common migraine.

Interestingly, these symptoms correspond to those of premenstrual syndrome (PMS). For many women, the premenstrual week *is* the week before the migraine, which often arrives on the day before menstruation, or on the first or second day of the period.

A common migraine attack may last for three or four days, as compared to the classical migraine's duration of several hours. Whereas in the classical migraine, the pain is frequently concentrated in one area, common migraineurs often feel their pain spreading throughout their head, face, and jaw, and sometimes even to the back of their head and neck.

With these migraines as with classical migraines, nausea, vomiting, diarrhea, and increased urination are common. The nausea may be due to an oversensitivity to odors, or to chemical substances circulating throughout the body. Sometimes people with these migraines will feel abdominal pain, as well.

Common migraineurs also display extreme sensitivity to light (*photophobia*) and to sound (*sonophobia*). They may get a mild fever during their headaches. Sometimes they have periods of fainting, whether from the pain or from other brain disturbances is unclear.

OTHER TYPES OF MIGRAINE

ICE PICK HEADACHES

This type of headache is experienced as jabs and jolts of brief, piercing pain to various locations around the head. It may occur frequently, or only occasionally. When it does occur, the attack lasts from seconds to minutes.

This type of headache is a migraine variant. Usually, it remits (stops for an unspecified length of time) spontaneously. However, it should be reported to your doctor, so that he or she can investigate more fully. Such headaches are effectively treated with indomethacin, an anti-inflammatory medication.

BENIGN EXERTIONAL HEADACHE

This type of headache is brought on by some mild exertion, such as coughing, sneezing, stooping, bending, or straining. Like the ice pick headache, it's a migraine variant that may last only briefly, although this type of headache may also last up to several hours. It's called "benign" because it is not life threatening, but it, too, should be reported to your physician, who may choose to treat it with indomethacin.

MIGRAINE PATTERNS AND PERSONALITIES

Many people are aware of patterns with their migraines. Others discover a pattern when they begin to keep a headache diary, as we recommended in Chapter 1. If you see a pattern to your headaches, you will be able to focus more effectively on changing the things in your life that are setting off the migraine pain.

MENSTRUAL MIGRAINES

One common migraine pattern is to get headaches around the time of the menstrual period. Migraineurs who

fit this pattern may have to be extra careful to avoid food
that may set off migraines at this time. They may find that
alcoholic beverages are certain to cause headaches then,
whereas they are less vulnerable at other times. Likewise,
stressful situations may trigger headaches around this time
far more than at any other. (For more on menstrual migraines, see Chapter 8.)

WEEKEND MIGRAINES

Another common migraine pattern is the weekend migraine. There are many different theories about why this
happens. Some say that changing one's sleep pattern brings
on a migraine. They recommend that migraineurs wake up
at the same time every day, even if they then go back to
sleep.

Others attribute weekend migraines to changes in diet
—less caffeine, more sugar and sweet foods. (For suggestions on how to treat migraine through diet, see Chapter 7.)

Still others relate weekend migraines to the migraineur's handling of stress. They suggest that migraineurs
tend to handle stress extremely well—but then get headaches *afterwards*. They're particularly vulnerable to migraine after stress is over due to the lowered levels of
"stress chemicals" in their bodies (noradrenaline, steroids,
etc.). (If this image of rising to a stressful occasion followed
by a headache during "letdown" has resonance for you, we
recommend that you look at Chapters 5 and 6 for some
suggestions on coping differently with stress.)

MIGRAINE PERSONALITIES

For many years, doctors believed in the "migraine personality." People with migraines were supposed to be
rigid, perfectionist, and tidy. They were believed to be intelligent and hardworking, with a more than usual interest
in success and a greater than usual sensitivity to what others thought of them. They were also supposed to have difficulty expressing anger or other negative feelings, and to
suffer from overwork, excessive worry, resentment, and fatigue.

Now the concept of the migraine personality is far

more likely to be greeted with skepticism. Many people with so-called migraine personalities never get migraines (though they may get ulcers, fatigue, lower back pain, or other physical expressions of stress—or no physical disorders at all!), while many people who suffer from migraine don't fit the migraine personality.

In fact, scientists have even challenged the idea that poor handling of stress is the central cause of migraine. In a study of 100 migraineurs, over half had their first attack during a stressful time—but that left many more who did *not* have their first attack at a stressful time. Further, this study found no evidence that these migraineurs showed any more evidence of neurosis than people who didn't have migraines.

What may be true is that if you do have difficulty expressing anger or saying no to extra responsibility, you may be setting yourself up for emotional experiences that will trigger your biological vulnerability to migraine. Your headaches' ultimate *source* may be the biochemistry you were born with; your headaches' *triggers* may be related to your feelings about others and yourself.

Even here, however, diet and exercise have been shown to have a profound effect on these feelings, even without the addition of relaxation techniques or formal counseling. Once again, the mind and the body show themselves to be profoundly interrelated.

If you feel that your health care practitioner is incorrectly characterizing you as a migraine personality, you may wish to discuss the situation or consider finding another doctor. Or you may decide that there is some value in the insights. Once again, it's up to you to decide, based on your awareness of your mind and your body, plus the level of respect and trust you feel for your health care worker.

MIGRAINES AND HYPERTENSION

Hypertension, or high blood pressure, is more frequently found in migraineurs than in the population at large. Once again, however, we don't fully understand this relationship. It seems that, if blood pressure goes up too high, this may provoke increased headache. Yet some medications to combat hypertension (reserpine, hydralazine, diuretics) can themselves trigger headaches. On the other hand, certain drugs for high blood pressure, such as the beta blockers (Inderal) and the calcium channel blockers (Calan), are often very effective in preventing migraine. (For more on medication and headaches, see Chapter 3.)

Apparently, the increase of pressure within the skull can cause a headache. But the blood pressure as recorded in the arm would have to be extremely high, in the area of 200/140 (versus a normal blood pressure of 120/80) to cause a headache.

Hypertensive headaches—that is, headaches that can be related to an increase of blood pressure within the skull —usually begin in the back of the head. They often start in the early morning, or wake the person from sleep. They may be accompanied by nausea or vomiting.

If you have both migraines and hypertension, we strongly recommend reviewing your medication very carefully with your physician, so that you're aware of any possibility that medication for one syndrome may be making the other syndrome worse. (Again, for more details, see Chapter 3.) In our opinion, the best ways to combat both headaches and hypertension may or may not always include medication, but should always include diet, exercise, and relaxation techniques. If medication is necessary, be sure you know what possible side effects you may be experiencing, and work with your doctor on reducing or eliminating that medication as soon as it's safe to do so.

MIGRAINE TRIGGERS

As we've stated repeatedly, migraines are a biochemical event, probably caused by a central nervous system disorder. Migraines may be triggered by a variety of factors, however, both emotional and physical.

It's also true that headache triggers work differently at different times and under different circumstances. If your diet is high in sugar, caffeine, or alcohol, you may be far more susceptible to emotional triggers that would not affect you if you were on a different diet. If your headaches are related to your menstrual periods, alcohol, sugar, or stress may trigger a headache during the week before your period but be relatively "safe" during the week after.

We present the following information about headache triggers in order for you to further increase your body awareness. We recommend keeping a headache diary with these factors in mind, so that you can begin to identify patterns and feel what's likely to set off a headache for yourself.

Emotional Triggers

Stress, depression, frustration, or letdown may all trigger a migraine. The physical basis of this theory relates to the adrenaline that is released during stressful situations. Adrenaline is a neurotransmitter that stimulates the body to mobilize against danger, as though it had to be ready to "fight or take flight." One type of adrenaline, noradrenaline, stimulates blood vessels to constrict, so that blood will circulate through the body with greater force. Then, once the stressor is gone, hormone and neurotransmitter levels drop and blood vessels dilate. (For more details on this process, see pages 199–201 in Chapter 7.)

If you sense that emotional triggers are setting off your migraines, try not to use this information to make yourself feel guilty or self-critical. Recognize that your body is giving you information about what it needs: another way of responding to difficult, challenging, and exciting situations. Chapters 5 and 6 suggest a variety of psychological and physical suggestions that may assist you in changing your response.

Weather

Some migraineurs get headaches during certain kinds of weather: damp, cloudy days, or dry, windy days. Some people's headaches are set off by the hot, dry air of a sauna. Others are particularly sensitive to the so-called "ill winds," the Argentine zonda, the Mediterranean sirocco, the southern California Santa Ana, the Swiss foehn, the Greek maltemia, the Israeli sharav, the Sumatran bohorok, the French autun, and the hot, dry winds of the Arizona desert.

Interestingly, studies of nonmigraineurs who experienced the Israeli sharav showed that the change in weather actually affected people's biochemistry, in addition to the physical discomfort. Studies of the Israeli sharav and the Middle Eastern bora (cold, rainy weather) showed that many experienced symptoms remarkably similar to those of the premigraine period: malaise, irritability, depression, and a general feeling of weakness. These feelings seemed to correspond to altered levels of serotonin, thyroxin, and steroids, and to change in amine metabolism.

The source of these changes appears to be in the electrical charge of ions in the air. Ions are electrically charged particles, either positive or negative. Weather and air pollution affect the ratio of charged to uncharged particles, which seems in turn to affect people's propensity to headache. There's a greater concentration of ions in water, which may explain why some people find it restful to be near a lake or the ocean.

Migraineurs who are sensitive to the weather seem to react to changes in indoor and outdoor temperature, air-conditioning or the lack of air-conditioning, increased humidity, higher altitudes, and shifts in atmospheric pressure. Thus low pressure weather fronts, with their falling temperatures and rising humidity, are likely to trigger a migraine, as is the season of winter generally. Airplane rides may also set off migraines due to shifts in atmospheric pressure, as well as several other factors, such as excitement, foods, alcohol, and lack of sleep on a long flight.

Light

Some 30 percent of migraineurs get headaches from bright or flickering lights. Light somehow stimulates the excitability of a migraineur's brain. Relaxation techniques and diet may offer some protection. Wearing sunglasses and broad-brimmed hats are more immediate methods you might try.

ALTITUDE

Most migraineurs suffer more at higher altitudes, possibly because of the reduction of oxygen at these levels. The body tries to compensate for the lack of oxygen by dilating the blood vessels, so that more oxygenated blood can reach the brain and body. When the brain's blood vessels dilate, people develop headache.

Some people develop acute mountain sickness at 8000–12,000 feet, and develop severe headache as a result, including vomiting, lassitude, and insomnia. The treatment for such conditions is either descending 3000 feet, inhaling pure oxygen, or taking the medications Diamox or steroids.

Exercise may improve circulation and breathing, so that blood is more oxygenated and travels more evenly throughout the body. Vitamin C may also be useful for this condition.

MOTION

For reasons we don't completely understand, the motion of traveling on a train, bus, boat, or car may set off a migraine. Children who eventually get migraines may begin by suffering from motion sickness for several years before headaches begin.

SLEEP CHANGES

As we've seen, some migraineurs wake up out of a sound sleep with headaches. Others get headaches from sleeping more or less than usual, or routinely wake up with a headache. Changes in the sleep-wake cycle often trigger migraines.

Researchers speculate that migraines are related to the REM phase of sleep. REM stands for "rapid eye movement," the period of sleep in which dreaming occurs. Along with rapid eye movement beneath closed lids, this period of sleep is characterized by lower electrical voltage of brain activity, higher frequency brain waves as measured by the EEG, a faster heartbeat, more rapid breathing, and consequently, more blood to the brain.

Possibly this change in brain and body function triggers a migraine. It's also possible that the emotional effects of dreaming set off stress and headache pain. Other chemical changes may take place at this time, which we know is essential to mental health and well-being.

If sleep changes seem to trigger your migraines, try to regularize your sleeping patterns as much as possible. Aerobic exercise may also combat the pattern of waking up with a headache, as may relaxation techniques practiced during the day and before bedtime.

MIXED HEADACHES

A new pattern of headaches that doctors have recently come to recognize is known as "mixed headaches." Mixed headaches are various combinations of muscle contraction headaches and migraine. Often, a person who has suffered for years from one type of headache will begin to experience some combination, providing still further evidence for the hypothesis that both muscle contraction headaches and migraines have a common source in a central nervous system disorder.

We've already discussed the mixed headache where a migraineur will develop a muscle contraction as well, possibly due to bracing the muscles against the pain, or stiffening neck and shoulder muscles in an effort to keep from moving the head. There are two other patterns of mixed headache.

One is when a person who basically has muscle contraction headaches occasionally develops migraine symptoms as well. These may include sensitivity to light, difficulties with the digestive system (including nausea and possibly vomiting), and some blood vessel changes.

The other pattern is known as chronic daily headache. It occurs when a migraineur begins to get a near-constant headache. A person with occasional migraines develops near-constant muscle contraction headaches. The migraines may come once or twice a week, or less than once a month. The pain of the "constant" headache is a steady, squeezing, band-like sensation that doesn't seem to be located in any specific area.

The transition usually takes place in one's thirties or forties. One study of some 515 chronic daily headache patients showed that most began with occasional migraines but had developed daily chronic headaches within eight to ten years later. This pattern has been called "evolutive migraine."

This syndrome is usually accompanied by an overuse of pain-relieving medication, depression, anxiety, and sleep disturbances. It generally occurs in people with a family history of headaches, and possibly a family history of depression and/or alcoholism as well. In the study of 515 patients, there was a higher than expected incidence of substance abuse, alcoholism, and depression among the patients themselves. Some 77 percent of those patients were taking pain relievers every day. (For more on the effects of taking daily pain relievers, see the section on "The Analgesic Rebound Effect" in Chapter 3.)

The central biochemical disorder at the root of this condition seems to have something to do with disturbances of the amine system, the set of chemicals that act within the brain as neurotransmitters, carrying messages of pain and other sensory experience from one brain cell to the next. Possibly the disorder involves the underproduction of endorphins, the body's natural pain reliever, an underproduction that is compounded by the overuse of taking "artificial" pain relievers. Another theory is that mixed headaches are caused by a disturbance of either the brain stem or the hypothalamus, the organ that regulates sleep patterns, appetite, and other body rhythms.

CLUSTER HEADACHES

Cluster headaches have the dubious distinction of being the most painful type of headache there is. Patients interviewed about these headaches say that the pain is far worse than complicated childbirth or accidental amputation.

These headaches affect less than 1 percent of the population, and they are frequently misdiagnosed. Because their symptoms include a runny or stuffed nostril and watering eye on the same side of the head that the pain is felt, they are often mistakenly thought of as sinus related, or due to allergies. In fact, they are another type of vascular headache, in which the pain may be related to the constriction and then dilation of blood vessels around the head, especially the carotid artery.

Unlike migraines, which are more common among women, cluster headaches are more common among men, to a ratio of 5 or 6 to 1.

If your headaches are short, severe attacks of eye pain, lasting about thirty to ninety minutes, with a pain so intense that you are almost literally suicidal, you may be suffering from cluster headaches. Other symptoms of cluster headaches include a drooping eyelid, red eye, small pupil, running nostril, and tearing eye, all on the side of the pain, which has been described as a hot poker being thrust into the eye, or as a stabbing, pushing force that penetrates the head.

Three Types of Cluster Headache

The most frequent type of cluster headache is the episodic cluster. Some 80 to 90 percent of cluster sufferers have this type of headache. For a period of four to six weeks, a person may get from one to three headaches a day. This is followed by a headache-free period of remission, lasting from more than five months, usually, up to one year or more.

In the subchronic cluster pattern, the remissions last less than six months. In the chronic cluster pattern, people experience no remission for at least a year, getting headaches several times a week during that time, up to three per day.

Symptoms of a Cluster Headache

As one patient describes, a cluster headache may be heralded with an elated, energetic feeling. Then there's a sense of fullness in the ear on one side, as when one descends in an elevator. After that, a sense of dull discomfort indicates that the attack is about to begin. This preliminary phase of discomfort usually lasts less than five minutes.

When the pain comes, it becomes progressively more severe. It always occurs on one side of the head only. One cluster sufferer described his experience as first a stabbing pain, then a spreading crescent of pain, then pain translated into a narrow, intense force, pushing through the head, as the headache peaks. About 70 percent of the time, this pain is nonthrobbing.

Usually the pain begins in the gum, cheek, temple, forehead, eye, or all over one side of the head. However, it may be felt in the lower face or around the jaw. This sometimes leads to a misdiagnosis of cluster headaches as a dental problem.

While the headache lasts, the nostril stuffs, then runs and the eye turns red. Most people can't sit still because the pain is so intense. They may scream aloud in agony, rock, pace, or literally bang their heads against the wall, trying to stop the pain. Eventually, the headache peaks, the headache events repeat themselves in reverse order, and the headache ends.

Cluster headaches usually last about ninety minutes, but the range is from twenty minutes to three hours. The most common times of day to get cluster headaches is between 6 P.M. and 8 P.M., which may be related either to the end of the working day, or to the end of daylight; and ninety minutes after sleep begins, when the first episode of REM sleep has begun. It's also common to get cluster headaches during later periods of REM sleep. The headache pain then wakes the person from sleep early in the morning.

Cluster headaches usually begin after the age of twenty. The episodic pattern tends to last an average of two months, with a one- to three-month range, during which the person may get from two attacks per week to ten per day. Then there's a remission, from six to twenty-four months, with an average length of one year.

In about 10 percent of people who get cluster headaches, the length of the cycle lengthens until the person is getting almost daily attacks for a period that lasts months, or even years. Sometimes this switch from short cluster cycles to long ones happens suddenly, without the gradual transition.

Chronic Paroxysmal Hemicrainia (CPH)

This is a type of headache that is like a cluster headache, but unlike clusters, is more common in women than in men. This apparent cluster variant may bring on up to fifteen brief attacks, each lasting ten to thirty minutes. Fortunately, it is especially responsive to indomethacin.

Causes of Cluster Headaches

As with other headaches, there's a lot we don't know about root causes. However, we do notice that cluster headaches seem to be tied to circadian rhythms (the body's rhythms of sleep and waking and its responses to daylight and darkness). Cluster patients seem to suffer from an alteration in the "biological clock"—one of the nuclei of the hypothalamus, an area deep within the brain near the pituitary gland. Available hours of daylight stimulate the pineal gland, which in turn communicates with the hypothalamus. Thus a change in available hours in daylight might set off a "chain reaction" that could trigger a headache.

It's common for headaches during the cluster cycle to occur twice a day, about twelve hours apart, or once a day, at the exact same time. This suggests that they are related to a disorder of the hypothalamus, the body's timekeeper.

This latter theory is supported by evidence that patients with episodic cluster headache usually get their cycles at the same time of year. In a study of 400 patients that included 900 headache cycles over a ten-year period, July and January turned up as the peak periods of cluster frequencies. As days got longer or shorter, cluster cycles began increasing in frequency, to a peak of the greatest number of cycles at seven to ten days after the longest or the shortest day of the year. The changes to Daylight Savings or Standard Time produced a decrease in the number of cluster cycles some seven to ten days after these changes. Sunlight cues somehow failed to stimulate these people's circannual pacemaker (the biological clock in the hypothalamus), which brought on the attacks.

The more immediate cause of cluster headaches may be vasodilation, the unnatural widening of the blood vessels. Or it may be related to an inflammation of or pressure on the nerves behind the eye, within a large vein called the cavernous sinus.

Since oxygen inhalation has been effective in treating cluster attacks, we speculate that a decrease in oxygen saturation in the blood may be somehow involved in bringing on the attacks. Or, possibly, oxygen is acting as a vasoconstrictor to the dilated blood vessel. Cluster attacks' tendency to appear during the REM phase of sleep, a time when the brain gets 65 to 90 percent less oxygen, supports these suggestions.

We haven't yet identified a cause-and-effect relationship between clusters and drinking or smoking cigarettes. But we would like to point out that there is a higher than usual incidence of these activities among cluster people. In one study, some 80 percent smoked and drank, and almost half the drinkers had more than two drinks a day. Other studies support the finding that cluster headache sufferers smoke and drink more heavily than others. However, stopping these activities didn't seem to help the headaches. Interestingly, cluster patients are extremely sensitive to alcohol while they are within the cluster cycle, whereas while not in the cycle, they can drink with impunity.

Depression and sleep disturbances are common during the cluster period. They may not be present during the remissions. This again suggests some involvement of brain chemistry related to these disorders, especially in the deep-seated structures such as the hypothalamus and the brain stem.

CLUSTER TRIGGERS

During the remission period, nothing will set off a cluster headache, except altitude on occasion. During the cluster cycle, however, air travel, high altitudes, strong sunlight, and even small amounts of alcohol will trigger an attack. So will "letdown" from periods of stress, as well as naps.

Other cluster triggers include exercise or exertion; foods with nitrites; medications that dilate the blood vessels, such as histamine and nitroglycerin, and certain heart and blood pressure medication.

Is There a Cluster Type?

Although we can't draw any connection between a "cluster type" and causes for the headaches, some interesting patterns have emerged. People with cluster headaches tend to be men with red, rugged faces and coarse, wrinkled, or textured skin, the type of skin known as *peau d'orange*, or "orange-peel skin." They tend to be taller than average, and the Caucasians tend to hazel eyes. They may have "thicker blood"—that is, blood higher in hemoglobin content—than other people.

Cluster types are usually gregarious, dynamic, extremely active and outgoing men, constantly on the go. They often do hard physical work or have jobs entailing great responsibility. As we've said, they usually smoke and drink alcohol and coffee to excess. Women with cluster headaches often have a masculine appearance and have quite atypical clinical profiles.

A sixty-five-year-old prominent Manhattan internist came to see us with a long-standing history of headache. He is an excellent physician and presented his own history, findings, and diagnoses. He gave a history of intermittent migraine attacks from age twenty-seven through age fifty-one.

At age fifty-one, he began experiencing different headaches from time to time. He described them as always on the left side of his head in the area of his eye and temple and told us they felt like a sledgehammer behind his eye. His attacks could last up to seventy-five minutes and were accompanied by a red and tearing eye on the side of the attacks. He would have several attacks in a twenty-four-hour period and would often pace to try and relieve his agony.

Although he had been successfully treated with several medications in the past, his headaches had now become so severe that he was forced to limit his own medical practice.

We initially put him on a program of Lithium and oxygen inhalation, and he was able to resume his professional life for four years without interference from headache.

Then major surgery triggered a recurrence of the cluster headaches, which we brought under control with verapamil, a calcium channel blocker. Although he is once again active, his case has shown us that cluster headaches may suddenly reappear in older men.

SINUS HEADACHES

Many people misinterpret their migraine or cluster headaches as sinus headaches. There is a condition known as sinus headache, but only about 2 percent of the population suffers from it. If your headaches are not accompanied by fever, running nose, and a general debilitation, they are almost certainly not sinus headaches, even though you may be experiencing sinus pain.

WHAT IS A SINUS HEADACHE?

Sinuses are air pockets within the bones of your nose, cheeks, and forehead. Mucous membranes line these pockets, secreting mucus, which is meant to flow through the sinuses down into the nose. Sometimes these passages are blocked. Then fluid builds up, causing pressure and pain in the sinuses. If the sinus membranes become inflamed, their blood vessels dilate, causing a sinus headache.

Infected sinuses cause pain around the eyes and/or across the cheeks and forehead. The pain is accompanied by nasal congestion and is constant and moderately severe. The headache lasts while the sinus is blocked and infected, and should disappear when the sinuses clear up. This usually takes about three weeks.

Many people have headache pain while their sinuses are blocked—and continue to have it after their sinuses are clear. This suggests that the headache is caused by some other factor, either muscle contraction or migraine.

CONFUSION ABOUT SINUS HEADACHES

When blood vessels dilate during a migraine, these may include vessels in the sinuses, so that pain happens to be felt there. This doesn't mean that the sinuses are in any way causing the headache.

Likewise, changes in weather, particularly low-pressure fronts, may bring on a migraine. This headache may be confused with a sinus headache, although again, sinus problems are not causing it.

A very dramatic headache pain with runny nose and tearing eyes might be a cluster headache, though these are even more rare than sinus headaches.

Interestingly, stress may cause a person to secrete mucus, which may then contribute to a sinus problem and/or a sinus headache. One study of people with sinus problems showed that when asked stressful questions, some secreted mucus, apparently in response.

HEADACHES, ALLERGIES, AND YOUR ENVIRONMENT

Occasionally an allergy will set off a headache that resembles a sinus headache, accompanied by runny nose, tearing eyes, and a sore throat. If you suspect that your headaches fit this category, be especially carefully in keeping a headache diary, so that you can identify the trigger that sets the headache off. Some likely food allergens are wheat, milk, and milk products. However, most food-triggered headaches are not due to allergies. (For more details, see Chapter 7.)

However, many people think that an adverse physical reaction is the same as an allergy. It isn't. You may get a headache from something you ate, or from fumes or vapors from, say, a cleaning fluid or a copying machine. This isn't necessarily an allergy. It only means that the substance has caused your blood vessels to dilate—a physiological reaction, but not an allergy.

If you think some element in your home or work environment is making you sick, see Chapter 9. There you'll find more information on possible headache triggers and ways to respond to them.

WHEN YOUR MOUTH AND JAW HURT: TMJ SYNDROME

This type of headache has its source in problems with the jaw, although pain may be referred to the forehead, ear, or temple. If you have difficulty opening your mouth or hear popping or cracking noises when you chew, you may have a malfunction of the temporomandibular joint.

The temporomandibular joint (TMJ) is the place where your lower jaw—your mandible—is attached to your right and left skull bones—the temporal bones. If you put your finger in front of your ear and move your mouth, you'll feel this joint.

If your headaches are caused by TMJ problems, this area will feel tender. Your headache pain will be felt as a dull ache or stabbing spasms, and you'll feel it in front of your ear, on your cheek, in your temples, or possibly in your neck and shoulder. TMJ syndrome is aggravated by eating and talking, as well as by grinding the teeth or clenching the jaws while awake or asleep.

Dentists believe that TMJ syndrome comes from mis-alignment of the teeth and jaw, so that the jaw muscles overcompensate. Possibly a weakness in the jaw is at fault. Stress and tension exaggerate an already strained area, compounding the problem.

Medical and dental treatment for this condition varies and may require a combination of strategies. Dentists may recommend a splint for the jaw to open the bite. Biofeed-back can be very helpful. You'll probably need to work with your health care practitioner to find the treatment approach that's right for you. Be careful: Some dentists may want to treat you for a TMJ problem, but the treatment may not always relieve the pain. Second opinions may be helpful for this condition.

EYESTRAIN HEADACHES

It's possible that your headaches may be caused by straining your eyes; that is, by contracting the muscles

around your eyes in order to see better. This muscle contraction may produce muscle contraction headaches, as the
muscles around the eyes interact with other muscles on the
face and scalp.

If you suspect this is the cause of your headaches,
check your eyes with an optometrist or ophthalmologist.
Make sure you keep your prescription up to date if you
wear contact lenses or glasses. Have a yearly test for glaucoma (a disease in which there is elevated pressure in the
eyeballs and the eyes film over), especially if you are over
forty.

If you wear contact lenses, keep your lenses clean and
free of protein buildup by means of enzyme cleaners. You
might check to see if you're allergic to anything in your eye
care solutions.

SEX HEADACHES

A condition known as benign orgasmic cephalgia produces a sudden, intense headache pain at the moment of
orgasm, lasting from several minutes to several hours. This
condition is more frequent among migraineurs than others,
but is not necessarily limited to them. It may also be related
to muscle contraction from the strain on the neck and shoulders during intercourse.

Usually, this condition doesn't indicate any life-threatening problem, although you should report it to your health
care practitioner to make sure this is the case. Certain tests
may need to be performed to exclude a serious cause of
headache, such as aneurysm or hemorrhage. You might also
want to consider whether there is a psychological dimen-
sion to this condition (for more details, see Chapter 5).

If, however, the pain from such a headache is incapacitating, you should be taken to an emergency room for
evaluation. If the condition persists, there are medications
that can help.

POSTTRAUMATIC HEADACHES

As the name suggests, a posttraumatic headache is one that results from a trauma, or injury, to the head, face, or neck. These headaches may come on days or even weeks after the actual accident, but more often immediately afterwards. Since they may involve fainting and life-threatening consequences, the sign of a headache pattern that may be related to an injury should be carefully noted and monitored for several weeks.

SYMPTOMS OF POSTTRAUMATIC HEADACHE

Symptoms of a headache caused by an injury tend to be fairly similar in kind, but do vary greatly in intensity. Interestingly, the intensity of symptoms doesn't seem to give much indication of the severity of the injury.

Post–head trauma syndrome is a term that covers all of the symptoms that may accompany posttraumatic headache, including dizziness, loss of memory, poor concentration, insomnia, reduced motivation, decreased interest in sex, ringing in the ears (tinnitus), blurred vision, and an inability to tolerate alcohol. Personality changes including mood changes and depression are also common. In about 10 percent of the cases, especially where there is dizziness, fainting also occurs. The symptoms may be made worse by exertion.

The signs of this type of headache usually come on within twenty-four to forty-eight hours after the injury, although sometimes there is more delay. If you are experiencing these symptoms, you should let your doctor know immediately, and be sure to have a friend or relative observing you, in case of fainting or falling into a stupor. Post-trauma symptoms may occur up to six months after the injury.

CAUSES OF POSTTRAUMATIC HEADACHE

Once again, we don't know exactly what causes this syndrome. One aspect of it is the possibility of the brain bruising when it collides with the skull due to a head blow or whiplash. Or the brain may absorb the energy of a blow to the skull, which causes it to vibrate.

This vibration or bruising may interfere with the activity of neurotransmitters, the chemical substances that carry messages among the brain cells. There may also be some interference in nerve connections within the brain caused by the sudden shearing forces of the rapid movement. This causes difficulties in making the mental connections required for concentration, thinking through problems, and carrying out daily tasks. The impact on neurotransmitters may be related to the personality changes and depression we have noted, since these substances are involved in biological depression and other personality disorders.

Whiplash (a sudden extension of the neck and head) or a blow to the head may also disturb the connections among muscles, nerves, tendons, and ligaments between the head and neck. It's also possible that the inner ear may be damaged, so that the brain is receiving incorrect signals about balance and body position. This produces the frequent sensations of spinning (vertigo) or dizziness.

Unfortunately, this syndrome is difficult to diagnose and doesn't show up in many ordinary diagnostic tests. Because head injuries, whiplash, and similar traumas are often the subject of lawsuits, doctors or others may cast doubt on a person's sincerity in reporting these apparently undetectable physical difficulties. These injuries are often real, however, and we urge you to find a doctor with whom you can work to identify and treat them.

Subdural Hematoma

This particular head injury is an accumulation of blood in one part of the head, due to a fall or a blow. The trauma leads the veins in the meninges to tear and leak blood between the layers of the meninges, the membranes that cover and protect the brain. The accumulated blood beneath the dura, or middle layer of the meninges, puts pressure on the brain, causing drowsiness, headache, paralysis, loss of vision, and eventually, death.

Such injuries are especially common among older people, whose veins are more fragile and who may also have a tendency to fall more often. Fortunately, subdural hematomas usually provide plenty of dramatic warning signs—but they still must be properly diagnosed.

The most common symptom is a persistent headache, which is likely to get worse as the days and weeks progress. Sleepiness, confusion, disturbances of vision such as blurring or double vision, nausea or vomiting, and weakness or numbness in one part of the body all suggest an injury of this kind. A skull x-ray can rarely detect a subdural hematoma; either a CAT scan or a process called magnetic resonance imaging (MRI) can rapidly show your doctor the cause of the problem.

WARNING SIGNS

If you or someone you know has received a blow to the head or neck, or has fallen and struck the head, watch closely for signs of a subdural hematoma for the next few days. Be aware, also, that such signs may show up months later.

If you suspect you are suffering from a posttraumatic injury, stay in close touch with your doctor, especially during the first few days. Don't take any pain relievers stronger than Tylenol, as they may cover up important signs of serious injury. Aspirin and other anti-inflammatory medication may increase your tendency to bleed, and so should be avoided. Someone should stay with you for the first day or two after the injury, and should wake you every few hours during the first night you've been hurt, to make sure you are still able to be alert and functioning.

If you faint or experience seizures, if you have a fever of 101 degrees or higher (a possible sign of brain damage), or if clear fluid or blood is coming out of your ears or nose (a possible sign of skull fracture), get to an emergency room. If other symptoms persist, make sure your doctor is aware of them.

BIOLOGICAL AND MEDICAL EFFECTS ON OUR EMOTIONS

We'd like to point out that depression—the feeling of being hopeless, despairing, and helpless to effect change—

may have biological as well as emotional roots. Viral infections, brain chemistry imbalances, glandular problems, nutritional deficiencies, some kinds of anemia, and hormonal imbalances may all lead to feelings of depression. Possibly there are other biological causes as well, having to do with root causes that we don't yet fully understand.

There are many medications—including some commonly used in headache treatment—that may create a feeling of depression. Drugs that reduce blood pressure, like the beta blockers; tranquilizers; and some birth control pills may all mimic biological causes of depression.

Having headaches may itself be a cause of depression, as we experience a major portion of our lives as painful and out of our control. This sense of losing control is itself a headache trigger, which in turn increases our depression. Even though biological causes, such as diet, may be the original reason for the headaches, the headaches take on an emotional life of their own after a while.

Thus we urge you to focus not on analyzing root causes, but on coping with the many facets of a headache's effect on your life. The secondary gains we spoke of may be your way of "making the best of a bad situation"; but they also may keep you from seeing some ways to make a bad situation into a good one. The depression that results from diet-induced headaches is still a psychological fact in your life, even though psychological "problems" were not the initial cause of the headache.

As we've said before, our minds, bodies, and emotions interact in complex ways. The good news about this is that any positive change in one area immediately has beneficial effects upon the others.

TRAVEL HEADACHES

Migraine sufferers are susceptible to headaches brought on by the stress and excitement of travel: disrupted sleep, time changes, and the specific problems of airline travel. These include eating foods high in salt, MSG, and preservatives; drinking alcohol; sitting in one position too long; and poor air quality.

Headaches can be avoided or minimized by planning ahead: take appropriate preventive medications before the flight; allow sufficient time to get to the airport; eat lightly and drink at least six glasses of water once on board. Walk about the plane frequently, but also try to get some rest in a comfortable position, and finally, take time to relax when you do reach your destination.

HOLIDAY HEADACHES

Holidays are a particularly difficult time for migraine sufferers who tend to overextend themselves. They shop and cook too much, skip meals, change their sleeping patterns, and attend smokey parties where they eat and drink the wrong things. All of this causes an increase in the normal pattern of headaches, which we refer to as the phenomenon of "holiday headaches."

We receive three times the usual number of phone calls in December and over three-day weekends and other holidays. To prevent or minimize "holiday headaches":

- drink eight glasses of water a day and avoid alcohol in excess
- don't skip meals and eat foods high in fructose such as tomatoes, grapes, and honey
- try to maintain regular sleeping hours
- don't overextend yourself physically, emotionally, or financially
- don't overmedicate yourself with pain medicine

OTHER MEDICAL CAUSES OF HEADACHE

Discussing every possible cause of headache is beyond the scope of this book. However, here is a list of possible conditions of which headache may be a side effect: infection; fever; constipation; neuralgia; carotodynia; temporal arteritis; stroke; meningitis; hypertension; a spinal tap; reaction to a toxin; side effects of medication or withdrawal from medication; reaction to alcohol, cocaine, or other recreational drugs.

[3]

DRUGS:
EFFECTS, EFFECTIVENESS,
AND SIDE EFFECTS

WHAT'S WRONG WITH DRUGS—
AND WHAT'S RIGHT WITH THEM

WE ALWAYS USE great caution and care in prescribing medications for our patients. On the one hand, we know that medications may have side effects, and in rare cases may even make headaches worse. On the other hand, we know that medications may offer a patient the first relief from headaches he or she has had for a long time. In some cases, medication may offer the breathing space to make other changes in headache patterns, or may offer a safety net to reassure a patient that there is a last-ditch defense against the pain. In other cases, especially for patients with chronic headache problems, medication is the cornerstone of our treatment.

Basically, medication has four major types of effect. It may elevate the pain threshold; that is, physical processes remain the same, but the person's experience of pain is blocked. It may modify muscle tone, causing tight muscles to relax or preventing them from contracting in certain ways. It may decrease inflammation of the brain, nerves, and blood vessels, encouraging them to constrict or dilate. It can also increase the availability of certain neurotransmitters and stimulate certain nerves to react, counteracting the usual biochemical processes that produce headaches.

All of these effects may be accomplished to some extent by drug-free methods, as described in the following four chapters on biofeedback, psychological approaches and relaxation techniques, exercise and massage, and diet. In general, the "side effects" of these techniques are overwhelmingly positive, while the side effects of most medication are at best only slightly annoying, though they can usually be dealt with by a change in dose or medication.

Ironically, when headache pain relievers are scientifically tested against placebos (pills with no pain relieving effect), up to 40 percent of the group taking placebos gets as much relief as those who are taking the actual medication. To us, this provides convincing evidence of the body's frequent ability to reduce and prevent headache pain without medication, as long as other methods are followed.

We are also cautious about prescribing medication because some headache remedies may cause depression, and/or addiction, conditions to which people with headaches have a particularly strong biological tendency. However, these conditions can usually be avoided, particularly in a strong doctor-patient relationship, when patients are responsibly reporting to the doctors and doctors are actively working with their patients to find just the right medication and dosage.

Thus, we and our patients sometimes decide that medication is the best solution at the time, even though our eventual goal is to find drugless methods of coping with headache. If you are using medication for your headaches, or if your doctor suggests that you do so, you need as much information as possible in order to make an informed decision about what treatment will work for you; to cooperate as fully as possible with the regime your doctor prescribes; and to monitor yourself for the effects of the medication so that you can work with your doctor in finding the best possible treatment. To this end, we provide the information in this chapter.

MEDICATION FOR SYMPTOMS VS. PREVENTIVE MEDICATION

There are two types of medication used to treat headaches. One type addresses the symptoms of the headache. It is taken just as the headache is beginning, or soon after it begins. Its goal is either to relieve the pain or nausea, or to reverse the physical process of the headache. The second type of medication is preventive and is taken daily to prevent headaches from occurring.

MEDICATION FOR SYMPTOMS

Medication for symptoms is most effective when headaches come no more than once or twice a week. Taking such medication more often opens you to the possibility of addiction, side effects, or to the chance that the medication may make your headaches worse. As we discuss in more detail below, pain relievers and ergot preparations may become so essential to your body that the lack of higher and higher dosages actually begins to trigger headaches.

The form of such medication is important: when taken in tablet form, the medication may take too long to be absorbed by the stomach and small intestine, so that it never reaches the bloodstream during the course of the headache. Apparently, even when the headache isn't accompanied by vomiting or stomach pain, something about the headache process may keep the gastrointestinal system from absorbing medication, even if the medication itself might be effective.

PREVENTIVE MEDICATION

Preventive medication is recommended when headaches come more than two or three times a month, when medication for symptoms doesn't seem to be working, or when people have medical conditions that would be made worse by some medication for symptoms. For example, people with heart disease, high blood pressure, and other blood vessel disorders should not use any form of ergot derivatives, since this medication works by constricting blood vessels and may cause chest pain and high blood pressure. People with peptic ulcers or aspirin-sensitive asthma, or who are using anticoagulant (blood-thinning) medication should not take any medication that contains aspirin. More information on these types of medication is available below.

Preventive medication is also recommended for people with a tendency to substance abuse, in order to prevent medication for symptoms from being overused.

VARIOUS TYPES OF DRUGS

OFF-THE-SHELF VS. PRESCRIPTION
Thirty or forty years ago, people tended to buy medication under supervision only. Even if their doctors didn't prescribe a medication, they usually had to ask a pharmacist for it, and thus came under their druggist's care. Today, it's possible to buy many headache remedies right off the shelf, without any medical professional's awareness whatsoever.

This easy availability of off-the-shelf drugs may lead people to be unaware that these nonprescription medications also have powerful side effects. In fact, off-the-shelf headache remedies may actually have a negative impact on your headaches!

Prescription medication is of course taken only under your doctor's orders. Still, many people don't realize the extent to which they themselves must be responsible for this medication, as well. It's important to follow the prescription directions closely (i.e., to take the medication in the amounts and at the times indicated), and to monitor yourself for side effects and to determine the general effectiveness of the medication.

Every individual has his or her own biochemistry. That means everyone will be affected by medication in a slightly different way. If your doctor is not readily available to discuss how your prescription drugs are affecting you, or doesn't seem interested in your perceptions, you might consider speaking to him or her, or finding another more receptive physician.

ANALGESICS

This category of medication is composed of pain relievers. They don't affect the physical process of a headache—
the muscle contraction or blood vessel dilation that leads
to pain. Rather, they affect the brain's processing of stimuli,
diminishing the experience of pain.

VASOACTIVE MEDICATIONS

This category of medication includes beta blockers,
calcium channel blockers, ergotamine tartrate, isometheptene mucate (Midrin), and some other medicines. They are
usually used for migraine or cluster headaches, since their
impact is to prevent blood vessels from overly constricting
(to start the migraine process) or dilating (to cause migraine
pain). Thus they tend to stabilize blood vessels.

ANTIDEPRESSANTS

The various antidepressants used to combat headache
are not usually given for psychological reasons—although
depression is frequently found to accompany headache.
However, antidepressants seem to be effective even when
depression isn't present, suggesting that they act on the
portion of the brain that triggers headaches as well as affecting mood or emotions. Most increase the brain's levels
of the neurotransmitters serotonin or noradrenaline.

TRANQUILIZERS

This type of drug may serve as a muscle relaxant and
antistress device, which may help decrease muscle contraction headaches and the migraines that are triggered by
stress. However, tranquilizers should rarely be used to treat
chronic headache disorders, and should not be used regularly.

OFF-THE-SHELF ANALGESICS

ASPIRIN

If there's one thing Americans are familiar with, it's
aspirin commercials. "Aspirin commercials give me head-

aches," sang humorist Allan Sherman over twenty years ago, and it's still true that in almost any randomly selected group of adults, you'd be hard-pressed to find even one person who was unable to quote a slogan from an advertisement for aspirin or some other related pain reliever.

TABLE 3.1

Major Ingredients in Off-the-Shelf Analgesics

	INGREDIENTS			
	ASPIRIN	ACETAMINOPHEN	CAFFEINE	OTHER
Advil				Ibuprofen 200 mg
Anacin	400 mg		32 mg	
Anacin (Max strength)	500 mg		32 mg	
Anacin II		325 mg		
Anacin II (Max strength)		500 mg		
Aspirin	300–325 mg			
Bayer Aspirin	325 mg			
Bayer Aspirin (8-hour time release)	625 mg			
Bayer Aspirin (Maximum)	500 mg			
Bayer Aspirin (Therapy)	325 mg			

(continued)

TABLE 3.1 *(continued)*
MAJOR INGREDIENTS IN OFF-THE-SHELF ANALGESICS

	ASPIRIN	ACETAMINOPHEN	CAFFEINE	OTHER
		INGREDIENTS		
BC-Powder	650 mg		32 mg	Salicylamide 195 mg
Bufferin	324 mg		48.6 mg	Aluminum glycinate
			97.2 mg	Magnesium carbonate
Cope	421 mg		32 mg	Magnesium hydroxide 50 mg + Aluminum hydroxide 25 mg
Datril		325 mg		
Datril E.S.		500 mg		
Ecotrin (Enteric coated)	325 mg			
Ecotrin (Max strength)	500 mg			
Empirin	325 mg			
Excedrin (Extra strength)	250 mg	250 mg	65 mg	
Excedrin PM	500 mg			Diphen-hydramine citrate 38 mg
Ibuprofen				Ibuprofen 200 mg
Medipren				Ibuprofen 200 mg
Midol	454 mg		32.4 mg	Cinnamedrine HCl 14.9 mg

| | INGREDIENTS | | | |
	ASPIRIN	ACETAMINOPHEN	CAFFEINE	OTHER
Motrin IB				Ibuprofen 200 mg
Nuprin				Ibuprofen 200 mg
Panadol		500 mg		
Percogesic		325 mg		Phenyl-tloxamine citrate 30 mg
Tylenol		325 mg		
Tylenol (Extra strength)		500 mg		
Vanquish	227 mg	194 mg	33 mg	Aluminum hydroxide 25 mg Magnesium hydroxide 50 mg

Reference: Robert W. Rosum, MS, RPH, Assistant Director of Pharmacy Services, Greenwich Hospital, Greenwich, CT 06830.

The numbers bear this out. In 1987, Americans bought $2.1 billion worth of off-the-shelf pain relievers. That accounts for more money than was spent on shampoo, deodorant, toothpaste, or any other single category of health and beauty product.

As a nation, we take more than 80 million aspirin tablets a day. As individuals, we average 100 aspirin tablets a year. That's 20,000 tons of aspirin a year, 16,000 tons of which are taken for headache. Add in all the nonaspirin analgesics available, like Tylenol and the various forms of ibuprofen (Advil, Nuprin), and you have at the very least a booming industry.

We've become so used to aspirin as a kind of headache cure-all—not to mention its other uses in lowering fever and easing arthritis—that it's worth taking a look at the history of analgesics (pain relievers). What was it like when aspirin was *not* a household word?

People had known for a long time that salicylic acid was useful in relieving pain. The problem was that this acid was so strong, it often induced vomiting and caused other stomach problems.

In 1896, Felix Hoffman, an employee of a German pharmaceutical house, discovered how to "acetylate" salicylic acid, producing acetylsalicylic acid—aspirin. This new drug *was* palatable—and within three years was put on the market by Hoffman's superior, Heinrich Dreser. (Dreser's other claim to fame was inventing a drug that he claimed was a useful alternative to the addictive morphine. He called his new drug "heroin.")

Aspirin skyrocketed to popularity as a headache medicine. It was first manufactured in the United States by its German parent company, Bayer, but competitors soon began fighting for their shares of the market. Since aspirin is basically aspirin, no matter how you package it, the competition took the form of advertising.

Thus, for example, Anacin was put on the market as a supposed alternative to aspirin. In fact, Anacin is actually just a mixture of aspirin plus caffeine. Because caffeine helps to constrict the blood vessels, increase the absorption of aspirin, and set into motion certain pain relief chemicals in the brain, it seems to help combat headache pain in some cases for some types of headaches.

Likewise, "extra-strength" aspirin is really just aspirin in a larger dose. No one has yet come up with a new formula for aspirin, per se, extra-strength or otherwise. Consumers seem to have a tendency to increase their dosage of aspirin from one to two tablets, no matter what the strength.

How Aspirin Works

As with many medications, the actual workings of aspirin are something of a mystery. We believe that it somehow affects the prostaglandins—lipid (fat) chemicals produced by the brain in response to constricted blood vessels, which in turn make the blood vessels dilate. Aspirin blocks the formation of prostaglandins by inhibiting an important chemical step in their synthesis. Thus aspirin keeps blood vessels from dilating, which in turn prevents headache pain as well as reducing inflammation of tissues and fever.

What we don't know is how aspirin raises our pain threshold. In many headaches, aspirin does not actually affect the headache process, but it does make the related pain easier to bear.

TYLENOL

Tylenol, the commercial name for acetaminophen, has a history that predates even that of aspirin. The drug was discovered by mistake in 1886, when an Alsatian pharmacist mistakenly filled a prescription with a mixture of vinegar and anilide. The accidental mixture brought down fevers and relieved headaches, but was not practical to use in that form.

Then, in 1889, the German chemist Karl Morner discovered that the body converts the vinegar-anilide mixture to acetaminophen. Soon Americans were treated to such whimsically named drugs as U-Re-Ka Headache Powders, "Funny-How Quick" Headache and Neuralgia Cure, and Telephone Headache Tablets.

These early versions of Tylenol were hard on the system, and they lost out to aspirin with little contest. Then, in 1951, McNeil Laboratories heard about another European version of the drug, which was used for children. First sold in a small red plastic fire truck, Children's Tylenol Elixir came on the market in 1955, and was marketed to adults as a prescription drug in 1974.

Soon Tylenol was competing with aspirin for off-the-shelf market shares as well. Television viewers were treated to all sorts of confusing, competing claims. These increased with the marketing of Datril, another acetaminophen product.

THE LATEST CONTENDER: IBUPROFEN

Ibuprofen, marketed as Advil and Nuprin, is the latest contender for the pain relief championship. Discovered in the early 1960s by a British researcher, ibuprofen is in the same biochemical class as aspirin—a nonsteroidal anti-inflammatory drug. However, it has a different chemical formula than its competitor.

Ibuprofen was first marketed in the United States in 1974 as Motrin, and expanded its activity in 1983 when another U.S. company acquired new rights to it from Britain. New products—and new ad wars—were the result.

How the Others Work

Acetaminophen (Tylenol) is not an anti-inflammatory drug. It does not seem to affect blood vessel activity, but does somehow affect our perception of pain. Ibuprofen (Advil, Nuprin), on the other hand, works in a very similar way to aspirin, since it is an anti-inflammatory drug and prostaglandin inhibitor.

The Relative Merits of These Drugs

It is true that aspirin has been effective in reducing many types of headache and other pain. On rare occasions, aspirin blocks migraine when taken early, and ibuprofen and related drugs are sometimes helpful at the start of a migraine. But all are virtually useless after the onset of migraines and cluster headaches. It's also true that Tylenol seems to have almost no ill effects on children, making it highly popular as a pediatric medicine.

Beyond that, it's quite difficult to evaluate the relative merits of the different drugs, let alone the relative merits of different brands. Some ads proclaim that Tylenol is prescribed more often by doctors in hospitals—but what they don't tell you is that Tylenol is provided to those hospitals at such low rates that it would be expensive *not* to use it.

The Federal Communications Commission (FCC) as well as the Food and Drug Administration (FDA) have been involved in various suits and claims of false advertising. Some have wondered why these government agencies don't simply run their own tests. We submit to properly test a headache medication, one must do a controlled study comparing an active drug to a placebo. In this way efficacy can be determined.

When it comes to off-the-shelf medications, perhaps the best rule to remember is to be aware that there are no chemical differences in the aspirin sold by the various aspirin products, including Anacin. Nor is there any chemical difference between the actual ibuprofen or acetaminophen sold by various companies.

However, there have been somewhat different side effects noted among the different drugs.

Side Effects: Aspirin

Aspirin may irritate the mucous membrane lining the digestive tract, producing gastrointestinal distress in 2 to 10 percent of the people who take it occasionally. Those who take large doses—ten tablets a day or more—experience marked gastric distress at the rate of 30 percent to 50 percent.

Aspirin is an anticoagulant and has antiplatelet effects. That is, it helps prevent the blood from clotting properly and thus can produce prolonged bleeding. This is what aggravates ulcers, as well as creating a host of other bleeding problems. Sometimes these are life-threatening. Sometimes these effects are less dramatic: for example, patients who frequently take aspirin may notice that they bruise easily.

Sometimes invisible (occult) blood can be found in the stool of people who take moderate to high doses of aspirin. This effect is especially important for menstruating women who lose blood vaginally and tend to be slightly anemic in any case. And two-thirds of those who regularly *over*use aspirin experience reduced red blood cell production.

Aspirin may also produce other gastrointestinal reactions. For example, people who are sensitive to aspirin may also be sensitive to foods that contain salicin (a chemical component of aspirin), foods like apples, oranges, and bananas. Likewise, processed foods and certain medications —those containing tartrazine dye, sodium benzoate, and iodide-containing agents—may also induce a reaction. These gastrointestinal problems may result in gastric ulcers, and may certainly aggravate peptic ulcers.

Some studies also suggest that aspirin stimulates the

pancreas to produce extra insulin, thus driving the body's blood sugar level down. In people with a tendency to hypoglycemia, this can produce the effects of dizziness, loss of concentration, irritability—and increased tendency to headache! (For more on the relationship between hypoglycemia and headache, see Chapter 7.)

Sometimes aspirin accumulates in the kidneys. Cumulative dosages may cause some kidney damage. This is particularly true when aspirin is combined with caffeine, as it is in some off-the-shelf medications.

Some people suffer from a form of asthma that is sensitive to aspirin. Middle-aged people generally may suffer from gasping, wheezing, or shortness of breath in response to taking aspirin. Some people suffer tinnitus, or ringing in the ears, as a result of aspirin's damage to their eighth nerve, the hearing nerve.

SIDE EFFECTS: TYLENOL (ACETAMINOPHEN)
The problem with Tylenol is that its unpleasant side effects are without visible symptoms. If you are experiencing problems from Tylenol, you may not be aware of it.

Like aspirin, the acetaminophen in Tylenol may accumulate in the kidneys, causing problems over time. Again, this is especially likely when acetaminophen is combined with caffeine, as it is in many off-the-shelf analgesics.

Too much Tylenol can cause liver damage, although this may be reversible if you take an antidote within eight to twenty-four hours. Patients who overdose on Tylenol can be spared liver damage in spite of toxic blood levels of Tylenol by taking Mucomyst (acetylcysteine). Interestingly, children are very resistant to Tylenol's effect on the liver, making Tylenol a drug that pediatricians rely upon.

Figures on Tylenol overdose are thus somewhat misleading. It's true that in 1987, as many as 14,500 people were treated in hospitals for acetaminophen overdose, as opposed to only 7700 for aspirin overdose; but most of these patients were children, who of course were being prescribed Tylenol in far greater numbers to begin with.

Unfortunately, because this drug has been on the market a relatively short time, and with relative ignorance of its dangers, we don't really know what its long-term side effects are. As with aspirin, it seems to be safe as an occasional pain reliever, but not a panacea that can be taken several times a week for headache pain.

One important note about acetaminophen: since it seems to be related to liver damage, it's especially unwise for heavy drinkers or heavy users of other medication to take it, since alcohol or drugs have already put a strain on their livers.

SIDE EFFECTS: IBUPROFEN

If little is known about the side effects of acetaminophen, even less is known about those of ibuprofen. Since it has some of the same characteristics as aspirin, it's probably best to assume that a sensitivity to one may indicate a sensitivity to the other.

We do know that some people react to ibuprofen with gastrointestinal bleeding or perforation, although ibuprofen does seem to cause less gastrointestinal distress than aspirin. Changes in vision are another possible side effect for some people.

You should be aware that higher doses of ibuprofen still require a prescription—so if you are taking more than four to six tablets in twenty-four hours, or if you are taking any amount of ibuprofen more than twice a week, you may be "prescribing" yourself an excessive dose. In addition, you may be programming yourself for the analgesic rebound effect (see below).

ASPIRIN AND HEART ATTACKS

A last word about aspirin: In 1988, the *New England Journal of Medicine* published the results of a study suggesting that the daily ingestion of aspirin would help prevent heart attacks. This study received a great deal of publicity, but less widely known was the fact that the study used a sample of relatively healthy doctors for its population. The study also found that aspirin might increase the likelihood of hemorrhagic stroke, or blood vessels bursting in the brain. Furthermore, a later study, smaller but with a longer-term time frame, found that aspirin actually had no effect on heart disease.

The final decision on aspirin and heart condition is not yet in. What is certain is that the dose of aspirin needed for the beneficial effect—if there is one—is very small. Aspirin in moderate doses relieves headaches; aspirin in minute doses—far smaller than those in your headache tablets—may help avoid first-time heart attacks in some people. This preventive effect results from 75 mg (the amount in one baby aspirin) of aspirin per day—but there are 325 mg of aspirin in regular aspirin tablets. A recent study suggests aspirin prevents recurrence of stroke.

SINUS HEADACHE REMEDIES AND OTHER OFF-THE-SHELF MEDICATIONS

Many off-the-shelf medications rely on a combination of aspirin or some other analgesic plus caffeine. (For more on the dangers of caffeine, especially for headache sufferers, see Chapter 7.) Then combine that with what you've read about the side effects of various analgesics. Extra-strength Excedrin, Cope, Midol, Vanquish, and maximum strength Anacin all contain a combination of an analgesic with caffeine.

Excedrin PM, Cope, Midol, and Percogesic contain an analgesic plus a mild sedative. The sedative does not affect the headache or pain in any way, and may create a mild addiction, causing you to develop headaches or other symptoms when you stop taking medication.

You may have been led to believe that your headaches are caused by sinus problems. Certainly the number of advertisements for sinus medication would encourage such a belief. In fact, sinus headaches account for only about 2 percent of all headache pain. (For more on sinus headaches, see Chapter 2.)

Sinus headache remedies are usually some combination of caffeine and/or decongestant plus an analgesic. In addition to the side effects of caffeine and the analgesic, the decongestant may increase your blood pressure or affect your circulation. Since blood pressure and circulation tend to be problem areas for people with headaches anyway, your medication may actually be making your condition worse. Besides, you may become dependent on this type of medication.

THE ANALGESIC REBOUND EFFECT

Perhaps most important for headache sufferers, relying too heavily on any analgesic may actually make your headaches worse. If your body comes to rely on an analgesic to achieve a state of normalcy—that is, no pain—it may actually produce headaches to signal its ever-increasing desire for larger doses. Analgesic rebound is the worsening of head pain secondary to excessive and chronic use of analgesic medication.

Many people abuse off-the-shelf analgesics, not realizing that these medications may have powerful effects on their bodies, even though they are sold without prescription. If you have daily headache and are taking analgesics every day, or even more than four days a week, you are probably suffering from the analgesic rebound effect. Far from easing your headache pain, the pills you are taking are actually making your headaches worse.

Studies on pain thresholds have shown that one regular aspirin tablet provides all the change in pain threshold that you are going to get. The medication will be absorbed in fifteen to thirty minutes, and will elevate your pain threshold for two to four hours. That's the most relief you are going to get. Taking more pills more often is not going to make any difference to your pain—except, perhaps, as a placebo effect.

A patient we'll call Mrs. Jones is a forty-three-year-old school teacher and mother of three who first began to have migraine at age twelve, the year she started to have her periods. They occurred one to two times per month for many years.

In her late twenties she began to have a mild headache all over her head which would last for several hours about two days a week. The pain was steady and nonthrobbing, and she would take two to four aspirin tablets to relieve it.

Over the next ten years her headaches became more severe and more frequent and her aspirin intake increased to five or six tablets per day. When the headaches became daily and severe, she started to use a medicine prescribed by her doctor which contained Tylenol and codeine. She began the rounds of doctors and by the time she arrived at our headache center, she had been seen by her general practitioner, an internist, two neurologists, and a headache specialist. She had been hospitalized twice and was given strong narcotics both times. Tests included a spinal tap, CAT scan, and EEG—and she had been tried on six different headache medicines.

After a three-hour evaluation by several people at our center, she and her husband were told that she had a combination of migraine, chronic muscle contraction headache, and analgesic rebound headache. She was gradually tapered off her headache medication after being admitted to the Greenwich Hospital inpatient headache unit for detoxification from the narcotics. An IV was started and she was given fluids, D.H.E. 45 to effect changes in serotonin transmission and constrict dilated blood vessels, and Decadron, a steroidal anti-inflammatory. She was taught biofeedback, given a new diet and specific physical therapy exercises for her neck muscles which were always sore and tender.

She left the hospital only seven days later on one medication at night to raise her brain's level of serotonin and given symptomatic medication to take if she developed a severe migraine. After a year and a half she is still doing very well, having only occasional headache and visiting us three times a year.

This kind of rebound effect can hold for aspirin, acetaminophen (Tylenol), and possibly ibuprofen (Advil, Nuprin), as well as for other off-the-shelf and prescription analgesics, including analgesics combined with caffeine, sleeping medication, and vasoconstrictors.

PRESCRIPTION ANALGESICS

Prescription analgesics tend to contain some of the same ingredients as off-the-shelf pain relievers, so what we've said in the previous section holds true for prescription medication as well. Essentially, prescription analgesics are composed of aspirin, acetaminophen, ibuprofen, or some combination, plus caffeine, codeine, and other narcotics, barbiturates, and/or an additional analgesic.

Most prescription analgesics are potentially addicting. Many contain substances that we believe to be liable to abuse. We've divided our discussion of prescription pain relievers into these two categories, but we caution you that either category may lead you to develop the analgesic rebound effect, and dependency on medication, and both categories may lead to side effects.

NONADDICTIVE PRESCRIPTION ANALGESICS

Parafon Forte includes acetaminophen and chlorzoxazone, a centrally acting muscle relaxant.

ADDICTING ANALGESICS

These include natural alkaloids, such as morphine and codeine, which dull the brain's ability to perceive pain. Or they may include derivative narcotics, as Dilaudid does, or synthetic narcotics, as Demerol does. As we've said, these substances all have the potential to become highly addictive.

Two of the most popular prescription headache analgesics are Darvon (propoxyphene) and Fiorinal. Darvon N includes aspirin and propoxyphene. Darvocet-N 100 contains acetaminophen and propoxyphene. Darvon itself is a derivative of methadone. It and the medications containing it are sold as nonaddictive drugs, but recent evidence suggests that they are addictive. In fact, we believe that Darvon may be no more effective than aspirin—and aspirin is certainly both cheaper and safer!

Fiorinal is also a combination brand name drug. In addition to aspirin, it includes caffeine and a barbiturate sedative (butalbital). It too has a high potential for abuse, due to the barbiturate. And, while it is often very effective, caffeine is not good in large amounts or frequently, as it can cause rebound headaches. Likewise, when used occasionally, and properly, Fiorinal is a very useful drug. The variant Fioricet contains acetaminophen in place of aspirin, for those who are aspirin sensitive or who get stomach problems from aspirin. These drugs can be used up to three days per week without rebound problems.

VASOCONSTRICTORS

A major category of medication used to treat migraine is the vasoconstrictors, the group of medicines that constrict the blood vessels. As you'll remember from Chapter 2, migraines have two phases: a preheadache phase in which blood vessels in the brain constrict (possibly causing the classical migraine's aura of visual and other disturbances); and the headache phase itself, during which overly dilated blood vessels in the scalp throb with pain. Vasoconstrictors are taken at the first sign of a headache. By keeping blood vessels at a normal level of constriction, they reduce pressure on the vessels' nerve endings and so prevent pain.

Ergotamine compounds come in four types: Sansert, ergotamine tartrate, D.H.E. 45, and ergonovine. These compounds, particularly ergotamine tartrate, are the most popular of the vasoconstrictors, and they have proven effective in granting relief of headache symptoms for many migraineurs. Other vasoconstrictors include isometheptene mucate (Midrin), phenylpropanolamine, and phenylephrine.

Ergot Compounds

Ergot compounds delivered by injection work in twenty to sixty minutes in 90 percent of the headache patients who use them. About 80 percent find equally fast relief in ergot delivered in rectal suppositories, and about 50 percent in tablets. It can also be inhaled or given under the tongue.

The mechanism by which ergot compounds work isn't fully understood, but we believe that they act upon the brain centers that regulate constriction of the arteries, as well as upon pain nerves carrying information to the brain. Ergot compounds also seem to act directly upon blood vessels. This medication is not to be used by people with high blood pressure, other blood vessel disease, or heart disease; people over 60; or people with some brain diseases like lupus.

Side Effects of Ergotamines

These include nausea, vomiting, and loss of pulses. We believe these effects result from the medication stimulating the part of the brain stem that induces nausea. The medication also has a direct effect on the blood vessel walls, which causes vasoconstriction.

In about 5 to 10 percent of those who use this medication, side effects include abdominal or chest pain, muscle cramps, vertigo or dizziness, or tingling in the limbs. If you are experiencing these side effects, bring them to your doctor's attention and work with your physician to find a more appropriate medication.

Dangers of Ergotamine tartrate

Because this medication is taken at the time of the headache, there's the potential for overuse. Some people react to certain high levels of this medication with a condition known as ergotism. Some of ergotamine's potential effects include cramps; chest pain; changes in the heart rate; and numbness, tingling, pallor, decreased pulses, or swelling in the extremities.

High levels of ergot compounds may also cause mental disturbances. Ergot comes from a rye fungus, and as early as 1670, we have reports of mental problems as well as gangrene resulting from peasants eating bad rye. Rotting rye is considered by some to have been at the root of hallucinations leading to charges of witchcraft in Salem.

Nowadays, we categorize ergot's most extreme side effects as hallucinations, mood disturbances, confusion, epileptic seizures, changes in vision, changes in temperature, and cramps, all possibly caused by reduced blood flow to the brain and other organs and its direct effect on brain chemistry.

Ergotism can be avoided by using ergot compounds in small doses no more than once or twice a week. It's easy to find increased uses of this drug "creeping up" on you, since your motivation for taking it is headache pain. But too frequent usage, even two to three times a week, can increase the frequency of migraine, known as ergotamine rebound headaches. If you suspect that you are overusing ergot compounds, start noting each use in your headache diary (see Chapter 1), and discuss your concerns with your doctor.

BELLERGAL

This antimigraine medication is a combination of ergotamine tartrate, an antinausea drug, and a barbiturate sedative. Many people find this combination quite powerful in combating their headaches. However, the combination is also a powerful one for creating the rebound effect, in which ever higher levels of the drug are needed to prevent headache, with an ultimate increase in the frequency of headache pain.

MIDRIN

Midrin contains a vasoconstrictor (isometheptene mucate), but no ergotamine. Instead, it has acetaminophen to ease the pain, plus dichloralphenazone, a mild sedative.

Midrin works on mild to moderate headache pain. It seems to cause less nausea than ergot compounds.

Side effects of Midrin include the feeling of being sedated or light-headed or dizzy, as well as the side effects of acetaminophen described above.

PREVENTIVE MEDICATION

Naturally, all preventive medication is by prescription only. We often use these medicines for patients with frequent or severe headaches. As patients improve, we lower the dosage and then turn to nonmedicinal methods. We find that preventive medication is especially useful for people who have or fear a tendency to become addicted to other medication, particularly among people who get more than one or two headaches a week.

BETA BLOCKERS

This type of medication prevents blood vessels from dilating. They have proven quite effective, but seem to have some side effects that may aggravate conditions found in headache sufferers, such as weight gain, increased cholesterol levels, depression, and tiredness, as well as the effects of hypoglycemia (see Chapter 7). These conditions may contribute physical and psychological factors to making headaches worse!

As with most headache medication, we don't know exactly how the beta blockers work. We do know that they somehow act on the brain centers that regulate blood vessels, as well as on the blood vessels themselves. In general, beta blockers have been significantly helpful to some migraineurs.

Inderal (propranolol) is the most popular of beta blockers. It's also used to treat angina pectoris, high blood pressure, arrhythmia, and tremor. It may lead to marked improvement in headache frequency, but will not cure the condition.

Other medications in this category include nadolol (Corgard), timolol (Tenormin), and metoprolol (Lopressor).

The dosage of this medication may vary quite a bit, as there are both long- and short-acting beta blockers. Your doctor may prescribe medication several times a day, or only once or twice. You should begin with a low dose and increase your use, depending on how you respond to the medication.

It's important to watch the dosage of any beta blockers you're taking. They tend to lose their effectiveness over time, requiring ever higher dosages. That's why, even when we prescribe this medication, we recommend that patients begin to employ other methods of coping with their headaches as well.

Some people should not be given beta blockers at all. These include those with certain kinds of severe heart or low blood pressure conditions, severe diabetes or hypoglycemia, and asthma or severe allergies with difficulties breathing. Suddenly ceasing to take the drug may cause increased heart rate (tachycardia) or changes in blood pressure, so it's important to taper off rather than quit cold turkey.

SIDE EFFECTS OF BETA BLOCKERS

These include a lower tolerance for exercise, fatigue, and weight gain. Some people experience a lower interest in sex, hair loss, and gastrointestinal distress. These effects are reversible when the drug is withdrawn, but the reversal process takes time, especially if you've been taking high doses of the drug.

Some people experience depression, loss of memory, or a reduced ability to concentrate when they take beta blockers. In order to respond to treatment of these conditions, they must stop or drastically reduce their levels of medication.

CALCIUM CHANNEL BLOCKERS

This type of medication works by preventing calcium ions from crossing the membranes of the muscle cells in the arterial wall. Restricting calcium ions in this way prevents vasoconstriction and spasms in the blood vessels, thus preventing the initial phase of migraine. This medication does *not* prevent other parts of the body from getting the calcium they need, and it does seem to help the conditions of angina pectoris, poor circulation, headache, and some stomach problems.

There are three major types of calcium channel blockers, so you and your physician may wish to experiment to see which type works best for you. These include verapamil (Calan, Isoptin), diltiazem (Cardizem), and nifedipine (Procardia).

Side effects of calcium channel blockers include a lowering of blood pressure, swelling ankles, dizziness, nausea, and constipation.

ANTIDEPRESSANTS

This medication is often effective in treating headache, even though it may not have any impact on the person's emotions. This suggests that the antidepressants affect the part of the brain that triggers the headaches. Of course, some migraineurs may also suffer from depression, perhaps for the same biological reason they suffer from headaches. In this case, antidepressants may be doubly effective.

There are several categories of antidepressants: tricyclics, monoamine oxidase (MAO) inhibitors, and tetracyclics. Fluoxetine HCl (Prozac) is in its own category.

Nortriptyline HCl (Pamelor) is preferred by some as it is less sedating.

One major tricyclic is amitriptyline HCl (Elavil, Endep). This medication has an impact on the part of the brain that regulates the experience of pain. It prevents the reabsorption of the neurotransmitter serotonin into the nerve terminals. This increases the concentration of serotonin in the brain, and prolongs its effects. In addition to regulating the brain's experience of pain, serotonin may help prevent depression and contribute to undisturbed sleep.

Other tricyclics include nortriptyline HCl (Aventyl, Pamelor) and doxepin HCl (Sinequan, Adapin). You and your doctor may wish to experiment with various forms of this medication to find the one that's right for you. A recently approved antidepressant is fluoxetine HCl (Prozac), which is reported to cause less weight gain as a side effect but can cause as well as relieve headache.

People who shouldn't use this medication are those with severe disturbances of heart rhythm or a recent heart attack, epilepsy, some forms of glaucoma, and enlargement of the prostate gland. If you are taking other sedatives, be sure to check with your doctor before taking these drugs.

Side effects of tricyclics may include lower blood pressure, weight gain, a dry mouth, trouble urinating, constipation, blurred vision, intense dreams, and a feeling of being sedated. In some cases, this drug will make glaucoma worse, and may aggravate prostate trouble. If a patient does get side effects, changing the dosage may alter them.

MAO inhibitors are the oldest type of antidepressant. They used to be difficult to take because they responded very badly in combination with certain dairy products and some other common foods. Now, however, in their newly available forms and dosages, they seem to be safer to take as long as the patient observes strict dietary rules.

Side effects of MAO inhibitors include lower or higher blood pressure, lower interest in sex, weight gain, difficulty sleeping, and dizziness. Some doctors think this medication is especially good for patients who also suffer from severe depression. Users must be maintained on a strict diet, avoiding tyramine as well as medications for pain or colds.

METHYSERGIDE MALEATE (SANSERT)

This is another type of medication used to prevent migraines. Some 50 to 60 percent of migraineurs who take it find it brings some relief. It seems to have some impact on brain action regarding serotonin and blood vessels. Methysergide seems to constrict blood vessels, and also works at serotonin receptor sites in the brain.

Side effects of methysergide include stomach pains, muscle aches, leg or chest pain, a swelling feeling in the chest or throat, difficulty sleeping, and possibly, hallucinations. Long-term use may create scar tissue (fibrosis) around certain organs and cause difficulties with blood circulation only correctable by surgery. Some doctors may feel that its use is justified. Clearly, you should be aware of all possible risks and benefits of this medication, and feel comfortable discussing them with your doctor.

Because of its effects, methysergide should only be used for three to four months at a time, alternating with two to four weeks when the medication is not used. During that two weeks, an electrocardiogram, chest x-ray and kidney x-ray (intravenous pyelogram, or IVP) or MRI scan and blood tests of kidney function should be administered to monitor this drug's effects. When the drug is stopped for the "holiday," it should not be ceased abruptly, but tapered off over several days or a week.

TRANQUILIZERS

Tranquilizers are one of the most dangerous ways of coping with headache. They may lower your motivation or ability to seek out and practice drugless ways of obtaining relief, as well as bringing other negative side effects into your life, including addiction, disorientation, loss of coordination, lack of concentration, drowsiness, weight gain, and, paradoxically, depression.

Some tranquilizers act as muscle relaxants, which may be temporarily helpful to those with muscle contraction headaches. Likewise, their apparent reduction of the impact of stress helps those with headaches triggered by stress. Migraineurs may benefit from short-term use of tranquilizers due to that medication's action on certain brain centers, reducing the possibility of headaches.

All in all, however, we do not recommend the use of tranquilizers to combat headache. Usually, there are many more effective ways of getting the same results. If you and your doctor decide that it's best for you to use tranquilizers, be sure you have a definite time limit in mind, and a specific plan for coping with the physical or emotional problems that led you to choose this method in the first place.

BENZODIAZEPINES (VALIUM, XANAX, TRANXENE, LIBRIUM, ATIVAN)

We believe that these tranquilizers tend to be addictive and must be used with extreme care. A benzodiazepine is prescribed to reduce anxiety, but it may increase depression, which is often also a problem for anxious people. Withdrawal from this medication may be especially difficult for such people, and may take a long time.

PHENOTHIAZINES (THORAZINE)

The tranquilizers in this class are even stronger than the benzodiazepines. This drug is used for schizophrenia, and is generally considered too strong for most headache treatments. However, those with a complicated biological and emotional history may find it useful. We use it in our hospital in-patient unit for those with occasional severe headache in lieu of narcotics.

Side effects of these tranquilizers include uncontrollable muscle reactions of the throat and tongue. With long use, a pattern of uncontrollable movements, known as tardive dyskinesia, may also appear, giving the person the sense that his or her muscles are acting "on their own." This spontaneous movement can continue for many years.

Thorazine may be of some use in cluster headaches. It can be used to help manage the pain, as well as to prevent nausea and vomiting in migraine.

OTHER PREVENTIVE MEDICATION

CYPROHEPTADINE (PERIACTIN)
This antimigraine medication is an antihistamine. It also acts at serotonin receptor sites in the brain, which affects the brain's perceptions of pain. Cyproheptadine is also like the calcium channel blockers, in that it prevents calcium from entering the cells of the muscles in the blood vessels, which helps prevent vessel spasms.

This drug seems to have fairly mild side effects, primarily the tendency to gain weight. It's an especially good medication for menstrual migraines, and is also helpful in combating headaches that may result in withdrawal from birth control pills (see Chapter 8). However, side effects do include an increased appetite, a dry mouth, and a sense of sleepiness.

We believe in giving cyproheptadine a one- to two-month trial. If the medication succeeds in bringing headaches down to one or less per month, it's usually possible to eliminate the medication altogether. We prescribe most of the medication to be taken before bedtime. This medication is also very helpful to children.

NONSTEROIDAL ANTI-INFLAMMATORY DRUGS (ANAPROX, MECLOMEN, MOTRIN, INDOCIN)
These are the medications used to combat arthritis. (For more on the relation between arthritis and headache, see Chapter 2.) Some people find these medications helpful in preventing their headaches. You and your doctor may wish to experiment with them. They can also be used to stop a headache.

Possible side effects include edema (swelling) and stomach pain. After prolonged use, this drug may accumulate in the kidneys, like aspirin. However, most people say they experience no ill effects from this medication. Be careful, though; these drugs can cause GI bleeding without warning in patients over sixty.

ANTICONVULSANTS
Such drugs as phenytoin (Dilantin), carbamazepine (Tegretol), and divalproex sodium (Depakote) are used to treat epilepsy. They are also effective in combating some

types of headaches, too. They are especially likely to be useful if your EEG (electroencephalogram) is abnormal. Such drugs may also work to combat a difficult headache syndrome when all else has failed.

TREATMENTS FOR CLUSTER HEADACHES

Cluster headaches are especially painful and dramatic attacks that seem to come in cycles, or "clusters." One of the best treatments for cluster attacks is the inhalation of pure oxygen, which seems to help many headache sufferers. (For more information on cluster headaches, see Chapter 2.)

SYMPTOMATIC MEDICATION FOR CLUSTER HEADACHES

Ergot compounds do seem to help cluster headaches within minutes, but because of the frequent appearance of cluster headaches during the cluster periods, sufferers may tend to overuse this helpful drug. Cluster patients don't seem to develop side effects like ergotism or rebound headaches from overuse of ergot compounds, as migraine patients do. Therefore, we do permit daily use of ergot compounds by cluster patients, even though we don't permit this to migraineurs.

Narcotics are not a good treatment for cluster headaches, because of the strong possibility of overuse. Similarly, oral analgesics are not recommended (in any case, they are not effective for cluster headaches). Some off-the-shelf sinus remedies do seem to have an impact, as they contain phenylpropanolamine, a vasoconstrictor, but you should not use these daily without consulting your doctor. In any case, breathing oxygen is the most effective and least dangerous treatment of cluster symptoms.

PREVENTIVE MEDICATION FOR CLUSTER HEADACHES

Preventive medication for clusters must be taken daily during the cluster cycle. Calcium channel blockers like verapamil HCl (Isoptin, Calan) and diltiazem (Cardizem) may be effective.

Methysergide maleate (Sansert) has been found to be effective for cluster headaches. It has the advantage of operating in a very short time.

PREDNISONE

Some 90 percent of cluster headaches can be prevented by prednisone, a cortisone-like steroid. This medication should not be taken for more than three to four weeks, but it is effective in treating short cluster cycles. It can sometimes cause the cluster cycle to go into remission.

Long-term side effects of prednisone include possibly lowered immunity against infection, weight gain, ulcers, hypertension, and diabetes, so you shouldn't be taking this medication for more than about twenty to thirty days at a time and never without medical supervision. We sometimes like to reserve it for people who are taking some time off from other medication, or for those who need to know that they have a foolproof method of relief when they are traveling or need a respite from a long, difficult bout of cluster pain. The most worrisome side effect is a serious joint problem called aseptic necrosis of bone, which fortunately is rare.

LITHIUM CARBONATE (ESKALITH, LITHOBID, LITHANE)

This type of medication has proved 60 percent effective in treating cluster headaches. It is most helpful in chronic cluster headaches. Lithium compounds are also used to treat manic-depressive states, a disorder that we believe results from an imbalance of some of the brain chemicals that may be involved in cluster and other headaches. Possibly the hypothalamus is implicated in both conditions as well.

Every individual responds to lithium differently, so work closely with your doctor if you are using this medication. Some doctors recommend a combination of lithium with calcium channel blockers.

Side effects of lithium compounds include nausea, vomiting, diarrhea, aggravation of skin conditions like psoriasis, unsteadiness, blurred vision, tremors, and possible stress on the thyroid and kidney. One must avoid dehydration, so people taking lithium compounds should not take diuretics or avoid salt, since this can increase the possible toxicity of the drug. During hot weather, you may need to take salt tablets to replace the salt you lose through perspiration.

OTHER CLUSTER TREATMENTS

Beta blockers, tranquilizers, and nonsteroidal anti-inflammatory drugs have all been used to treat cluster headaches, with very little success. Medication that desensitizes the body to histamines may also help. In unsuccessfully treated cases, cluster victims must be hospitalized. We've also noticed that cutting out smoking and drinking occasionally helps to reduce cluster headaches. Indocin, an anti-inflammatory drug, can sometimes be helpful in cluster headache. In-patient admission to a specialized headache unit can often be very helpful. In rare cases, a special form of surgery on the 5th cranial nerve may be effective.

TREATMENTS FOR MUSCLE CONTRACTION HEADACHES

Various types of medication may be effective in treating this type of headache. For pain that originates in the neck, nonsteroidal anti-inflammatory drugs may be helpful, including aspirin, indomethacin (Indocin), naproxen (Anaprox, Naprosyn), ibuprofen (Advil, Nuprin, Motrin), or meclofenimate (Meclomen).

Chronic tension headaches are often treated with tricyclic antidepressants, particularly amitriptyline HCl (Endep, Elavil). This medication is most effective for this use when taken in low doses at bedtime for several months. The dosage is gradually increased from 10 to about 50 mg given at bedtime. Nortiptyline HCl (Pamelor, Aventyl), desipramine HCl (Norpramin, Pertofrane), or doxepin HCl (Sinequan, Adapin) may also be used.

Beta and calcium channel blockers may act on the brain centers that produce the tendency to "daily headache," but these are less effective. Muscle relaxants may also be effective, such as carisoprodol (Soma), cyclobenzaprine (Flexeril), orphenadrine (Norflex), or metaxalone (Skelaxin). These should only be used on a short-term basis.

Some doctors prescribe tranquilizers for this type of headache, but as we've already explained, we don't. We'd recommend a definite plan for terminating the use of tranquilizers, with a specific deadline for ceasing to take them, if this medication must be used. Biofeedback training can be very helpful in treating muscle contraction headache patients.

TREATMENTS FOR POSTTRAUMATIC HEADACHES

Medication for posttraumatic headache must be prescribed carefully, since the brain has been traumatized and is not reacting normally. Tricyclic antidepressants may raise the brain's serotonin levels, helping the mind to reestablish many of the mental connections that the injury has disrupted. Various other medications, including beta and calcium channel blockers, methysergide, nonsteroidal anti-inflammatory drugs, ergot compounds, anticonvulsants, lithium, and various tranquilizers may also be prescribed.

However, you should be aware that any of these drugs may aggravate the mental changes produced by the injury. If these drugs affect your inner ear mechanism, you may feel an increased sense of dizziness as a result of taking them. In addition, of course, there are the usual side effects.

Sometimes nerve (neuralgic) pain is pinpointed and treated with a local anesthetic. In extreme cases, surgical intervention may be necessary. Biofeedback training can be helpful.

WHEN DRUGS DO MORE HARM THAN GOOD

Our own studies have shown that sometimes, if people with chronic daily headaches who are dependent on analgesics are treated by no other means than simply stopping analgesic medication, 50 percent of those who stop will do at least 50 percent better after the first month; and 85 percent will do at least 50 percent better after three months. This improvement occurs because the rebound effect we've been describing has been stopped; it's a striking indication of the need for caution in using pain medication.

If the medication you've been taking includes barbiturates, narcotics, tranquilizers, or sedatives, you may not be able to withdraw from it on your own. A doctor's supervision, or even hospitalization, may be needed. If you suffer from cardiac disease or hypertension, you will also need a doctor's supervision. In any case, it's generally best to withdraw from the above medication over a one- to two-week period under a doctor's supervision. Most withdrawal is safely and painlessly accomplished in a hospital headache unit setting.

Some medications, including over-the-counter analgesics, are quite difficult to stop taking, though withdrawal from these is in no way dangerous. The initial increase in headache pain may make this time quite trying. Sometimes Vitamin B_6 or the antihistamine cyproheptadine (Periactin) helps to ease this period. Midrin, antinausea medication, a mild sedative, or anti-inflammatory drugs may also be prescribed for this transition.

In one study we conducted, of sixty-nine women and twenty-one men who stopped taking analgesic medication, 82 percent had experienced at least two-thirds fewer headaches within four months. We believe that these results are definitely worth the difficult transition time, especially if you can work with your doctor to ease that period.

However, sometimes people feel helpless without their ritual of medicating themselves, particularly if pain has gotten worse. Cognitive/behavioral therapy principles, biofeedback training, or relaxation techniques may be helpful to cope with the psychological aspects of drug withdrawal. You can read more about these ideas in Chapter 4.

[4]

BIOFEEDBACK:
LEARNING TO
MONITOR YOURSELF

ONE ALTERNATIVE TO MEDICATION

IF YOU'VE READ the previous chapter and are concerned about using medication to combat your headaches, don't worry. There are lots of alternatives, many of which have their own *positive* side effects! It's also possible to combine these alternative methods with some use of medication, or to use these methods to make the transition away from using medication.

We cover these other methods—relaxation techniques, diet, and various types of exercises—in the next few chapters. We encourage you to look them over, so that you can pick and choose among many alternatives the ones that seem right for you.

One alternative that many people have found helpful is *biofeedback*, which is short for "biological feedback." It refers to a process whereby various machines give you feedback—or information—about some biological processes in your body. A machine measures the extent to which your scalp muscles are contracted, determines the circulation in your hands, or monitors the amount of blood pulsing through your temporal artery (the part of the external carotid artery that runs along the outside of your skull at the temple in front of your ear), or the arteries in your hands. As we saw in Chapter 2, this muscle contraction or blood flow is associated with headache. By receiving feedback about these processes, you can learn to modify them, to reduce or eliminate your headaches. Biofeedback is a scientific demonstration of the principle of "mind over matter," or, more accurately, of the complex interaction between your mind and your body.

HOW EFFECTIVE IS BIOFEEDBACK?

Various studies have found the biofeedback method to be extremely effective. One doctor found that it relieved 70 percent of the chronic muscle contraction headaches in those of his patients who had tried it. Other studies showed that biofeedback offered relief to up to 60 percent of the migraineurs who had used it.

Generally speaking, 50 to 70 percent of the people who use biofeedback get some benefit from it, whether in preventing headaches or in reducing the intensity or duration of headache pain.

BIOFEEDBACK FOR MIGRAINES

In one study of migraineurs, people in four groups received, respectively, either a combination of biofeedback and relaxation techniques, biofeedback or relaxation by itself, or a placebo. Some 65 percent of the group receiving the combination of biofeedback and relaxation techniques found some headache relief. That was compared to the 52 percent who found relief from biofeedback alone, the 53 percent who benefited from relaxation techniques alone— and the 17 percent that benefited from the placebo! (As you can see, "mind over matter" operates in some people even without benefit of other assistance!)

This benefit seemed to hold up over time. Follow-up studies of migraineurs showed from 57 to 70 percent improvement was still maintained some months or years after the initial treatment.

BIOFEEDBACK AND MUSCLE CONTRACTION HEADACHES

In a study of those with muscle contraction headaches, participants were again divided into four groups. Some 61 percent of those receiving biofeedback experienced some headache relief, as opposed to 59 percent of those using a combination of biofeedback and relaxation techniques, 59 percent of those using relaxation techniques alone, and 35 percent of those receiving placebos. (The placebos in this case were both medication—inactive pills—and psychological placebos—being given inaccurate data about their biofeedback experience.)

This is only one study, and the percentage of variations among the top three categories were very small. The data should not be interpreted to mean that biofeedback is clearly more effective than relaxation techniques, either alone or in combination with biofeedback. What is correct to interpret is that both biofeedback and relaxation techniques have been found effective by most people who suffer from headaches. We believe that if biofeedback and/or relaxation were further combined with improved diet and exercise, the number of those helped would be even greater.

BIOFEEDBACK AND CLUSTER HEADACHES

As we have seen, cluster headaches are somewhat more difficult to treat effectively than other types of headache. Unfortunately, biofeedback has been of only limited help. A few studies suggest that about one in four people with cluster headaches can reduce the occurrence of their headaches by biofeedback. We ourselves, however, have not found it to be helpful in preventing cluster headache and its benefit seems limited to helping patients cope with the pain.

BIOFEEDBACK AND POSTTRAUMATIC HEADACHES

There has not been any conclusive research done into the effectiveness of biofeedback for those with posttraumatic headache. However, in our experience, biofeedback is a useful and effective aid, especially if there is a component of muscle contraction headache present.

WHY DOES BIOFEEDBACK WORK?

The purpose of biofeedback is to bring awareness of biological functions into your conscious mind. The theory is that if your physiological functions are measured, and if you are aware of these measurements, you can learn to exert control over those functions.

Normally, we don't think of ourselves as being able to control the tensing of our muscles or the flow of blood to different parts of our bodies. Traditionally, we distinguish between *voluntary* processes—picking up a pencil, sitting down, opening our mouths to speak—and *involuntary* processes—breathing, the beating of our hearts, the blinking of our eyes. Voluntary processes require conscious thought and intervention. Involuntary processes continue whether we think about them or not.

Just because we don't have to think about a biological process doesn't mean that our minds don't affect it. As we saw in Chapter 1, we have lots of evidence of mind-body interaction from our daily lives. Think about a new love, an upcoming meeting, or a fight with your boss, and you may find your heart beating faster, your stomach contracting, or your palms sweating. In a sense, you have "controlled"— or at least affected—the involuntary processes of heartbeat, digestion, and perspiration.

Biofeedback focuses on the involuntary biological processes associated with migraine and muscle contraction headache. By giving you information about your body's condition, biofeedback helps you to become aware of these processes, and to modify them.

Biofeedback can also teach you how to achieve a physical state known as *deep relaxation*. This state apparently helps counteract the muscle contraction and uneven blood flow associated with headache.

DEEP RELAXATION: YOUR BODY AND YOUR BRAIN

When we say deep relaxation, we aren't talking about spending a quiet Saturday at home, or taking a pleasant trip to the beach. These experiences may be relaxing, but they don't necessarily produce the biological changes that deep relaxation refers to.

Deep relaxation is a measurable state of decontraction —looseness—in one's muscles, and a stable, even flow of blood to all parts of the body. Loose muscles and a stable blood flow are the opposite of the conditions that have been associated with migraine and muscle tension headaches.

Deep relaxation can be measured through checking the electrical energy generated by your muscles—the tighter the muscle, the more electric energy is produced. It's also possible to measure how evenly blood is flowing through certain arteries. These measurements are the basis of biofeedback.

There's another important indicator of deep relaxation: the type of electrical energy generated by your brain. Scientists have identified four types of brain activity: alpha, beta, delta, and theta. Each type of activity corresponds to a different frequency of your brain waves. The waves that your brain produces at the rate of between 8 and 13 cycles per second are known as alpha waves. Beta waves have a frequency of 13 to 30 cycles per second. Theta, on the other hand, has a frequency of 4 to 8 cycles per second, while delta waves come at the rate of 1 to 4 cycles per second.

It was once thought that these four types of brain waves simply corresponded to different states of the brain: waking, resting, sleeping, and deep sleep. Then, in the 1960s, Western scientists discovered that people could also exercise conscious control to bring about one state or another. This, of course, was an insight that many Eastern cultures had already discovered. Meditation, an ancient practice in Buddhism, Hinduism, and other Eastern religions, can be scientifically described as a technique for getting one's brain to switch from one type of wave to another.

As you might expect, this idea was greeted with some skepticism by the medical community. With the development of the electroencephalograph (EEG), however, we were able to find scientific data to further explain the process. The EEG measures the electrical waves produced by the brain, as recorded from the scalp. EEG measurements supported the idea that people could vary the electrical activity of their brains by various techniques. Today, computers accurately analyze the amounts and voltages of the different categories of brain waves.

DEEP RELAXATION AND THE
TREATMENT OF HEADACHES

As early as 1929, Dr. Edmund Jacobson had used his own version of progressive muscle relaxation to treat muscle contraction headache. By the early 1970s, we were getting the first reports on using relaxation and related methods to treat migraine. It seemed that deep relaxation helped counteract the muscle contraction and the unstable blood flow related to both types of headaches.

In 1969, we got the first description of a clinical instrument that could give feedback on various headache-related processes. The foundation for biofeedback had been laid.

At first, some of the members of the medical community were rather suspicious of biofeedback. In some circles, this technique was seen as a jazzed-up version of pseudoscientific theories about meditation, macrobiotics, and self-healing. But, as we have seen, the scientific benefits of biofeedback were undeniable. As we learned more about the potential negative side effects of medication, biofeedback became even more attractive. Ironically, the acceptance of biofeedback has now created even more openness in the medical community to other holistic, nonmedicinal methods, particularly techniques for achieving deep relaxation.

THE BIOLOGICAL BASIS FOR BIOFEEDBACK

BIOFEEDBACK AND MUSCLE TENSION

As we saw in Chapter 2, muscle contraction is often related to headache pain. We used to believe that this relationship only existed in so-called "tension" headaches. Now we believe that muscle contraction is present in both tension headaches and migraines.

We don't know exactly how this relationship works. Nor do we completely understand why, in some people, a certain level of muscle contraction is associated with severe headache pain, while in others, the same level of contraction is not associated with pain at all. As we saw in Chapter 2, we once believed that muscle contraction somehow "caused" headache pain, whereas we now suspect that some biochemical or nervous system disorder may cause both the muscle contraction and the related pain. In fact, current theories hold that chemical messengers in the brain, particularly serotonin, may not be functioning properly in people with headache. This malfunction may in itself be enough to produce pain in spite of the fact that levels of muscle tension are normal.

Even though we don't fully understand what causes muscle contraction headaches, it does seem to be true that relaxing certain muscles helps to prevent and/or reduce some types of headache pain. Contracted muscles create toxic by-products, such as lactic acid, which may contribute to the pain we feel when a muscle is contracted for a long period of time. Contracted muscles also reduce the flow of blood and oxygen to the muscles' area.

Chronic muscle tension can be maintained by a reflex between the muscle fibers and the spinal cord. This reflex must be "reset" at a lower level in headache sufferers, so that muscles are relaxed, rather than tensed. Resetting this reflex can be done through achieving the state of deep relaxation. Biofeedback training can teach people how to achieve this state.

BIOFEEDBACK AND BLOOD FLOW

As we saw in Chapter 2, we once believed that only migraine headaches were related to blood flow. Now we believe that both migraine and muscle contraction headaches are related to problems with circulation.

In muscle contraction headaches, as we have seen, contracted muscles mean a reduced blood flow to the affected area. In migraine headaches, blood flow through certain vessels tends to vary more and more during the three days or so before the headache begins. There is some evidence that migraines are preceded by a decreased blood flow to certain areas of the brain. Then, during the throbbing, painful period of the migraine, there is an expansion and swelling of the blood vessels outside the brain, such as in the temple. In both migraine and muscle contraction headaches, regulating the blood flow seems to reduce and prevent headache pain.

Once again, deep relaxation proves to be useful. It stabilizes the flow of blood to the brain, as well as to the constricted blood vessels of the neck and scalp muscles involved in muscle contraction headache. Deep relaxation also may decrease the flow of blood to some vessels, helping to prevent migraine.

BIOFEEDBACK AND HEADACHE PAIN

We've seen how achieving deep relaxation can help prevent headache pain. But what about when you're in the throes of the headache itself? Can deep relaxation do anything for you then?

Apparently, the answer is yes. Sometimes achieving a state of deep relaxation can stabilize blood flow, relax key muscles, and actually make headache pain go away. Moreover, doctors and biofeedback therapists have found that even when deep relaxation doesn't reduce pain, it can help you cope with that pain much more effectively.

The reasons for this throw still more light on the complicated interaction between mind and body. Getting a headache is a distressing emotional experience, as well as a physically painful one. You feel yourself to be completely disabled by something that is outside of your control. You may feel frightened, angry, panicked, frustrated, or depressed. These feelings may well carry over past the headache, as you contemplate your inability to do anything about a recurring event that disrupts your life.

If you know how to achieve deep relaxation, however, you may feel far less victimized and panicked by your brain. Instead of waiting passively for the headache to interrupt your life, there is something you can do. At the very least, you're distracted from the suffering; at best you may actually bring yourself relief. Instead of focusing on how badly your head hurts, you can concentrate on relaxing your muscles, regulating your blood flow, and achieving a state of calm.

Interestingly, belief in the ability to control one's headaches seems to be beneficial in itself, even if the belief isn't founded on anything more substantial than a researcher's comments. In one study, a group of people were told that they had successfully achieved deep relaxation through biofeedback techniques, whether this was actually true or not. A second group was told that they were unsuccessful, regardless of the facts. Some 53 percent of the group that had been told they were successful achieved improvement with their headaches, as opposed to only 26 percent of the group who had been told that they were unsuccessful.

That study produced another striking conclusion: people's *belief* in their bodily control was apparently a better predictor for headache relief than their actual ability to achieve that control. In fact, some people who actually *increased* their muscle tension while practicing biofeedback nevertheless achieved dramatic relief from headaches, apparently because they had been told that their muscle tension had decreased. The belief in their ability to cure their headaches was more important than anything about their actual physical state.

These results convey a dramatic sense of the kind of mind-body relationship that is possible for human beings, the extent to which we can heal ourselves if we only believe that we can. The scientific foundation of this result may be that belief in one's control of a situation causes the adrenal glands to release fever catecholamines into the bloodstream. As we saw in Chapter 2, catecholamines are released during the "fight or flight" reaction, when a person believes that he or she is facing danger. Catecholamines are neurochemicals that affect the sympathetic nervous system, and may thereby affect blood vessel size, blood pressure, muscle tension, heart rate, and the sweat glands. The release of catecholamines may trigger headaches in certain people if the blood pressure goes too high. However, a constant level of catecholamines may prevent vasodilation and therefore, migraine.

One type of danger that people perceive is the danger of having an uncontrollable headache. Thus, if one believes that headaches can be controlled, they are no longer a danger. "Fight or flight" is no longer necessary, and catecholamines are not suddenly released in large amounts. In such cases, even though other physical contributors to a headache are present, the headache may not occur.

BIOFEEDBACK IN YOUR LIFE

As you can see, gaining a sense of control over one's life and finding effective ways of coping with stress are generally beneficial to people who suffer from headaches —and to people in general! We deal more with these issues in Chapter 5. Here, let us repeat that a key part of biofeedback is becoming aware of the stressors in your life and learning new ways to respond to them. It also means becoming aware of your typical postures and movements, and learning whether these contribute to muscle contraction, which in turn may impede blood flow.

As we have seen, people with headaches are not necessarily less able to deal with stress than other people. Rather, they have a particular biochemical or nervous disorder that translates their stress more easily into headaches. (Other people may translate *their* stress into stomach disorders, fatigue, or lower back pain, depending on their biochemical or nervous makeup.)

Biofeedback can help you retrain your physiological system's responses to the environment. It can also help you overcome a possible genetic tendency to translate stress into headaches. But this retraining depends on your own awareness. The more sensitive you are to your own responses to stress, the more you can draw on your new ability to modify those responses.

Up to this point, we've been talking about biofeedback as though it were simply a technique. Perhaps it would be more accurate to speak of it as an opening, an opportunity, a new chance to experience the intimate connection between your mind and your body. Biofeedback is not simply a treatment that you receive, in place of or in addition to medication. Rather, it's a training that you can bring into your life.

THE MECHANICS OF BIOFEEDBACK

YOUR INITIAL VISIT

Biofeedback is practiced by a trained therapist. The biofeedback therapist's job is to train you in relaxation techniques and body awareness, with the aid of the various biofeedback machines.

Because biofeedback is part of a comprehensive approach to mind and body, the therapist is likely to begin by giving you a detailed questionnaire, about both your headaches and your general health. You'll probably be asked questions about the nature of your headache pain (Is it throbbing or pressing? Does it change during the headache or remain the same?), how long your headaches usually last, how often you get them, and whether you have any accompanying conditions, such as nausea, blurred vision, or numbness.

You'll also be asked about your general health history, about the medications you take for headache and for other conditions, and about your general diet and exercise habits. Some questionnaires may also include questions about areas you find stressful: work habits, family life, and other possible sources of stress (for our own questionnaire, see page 267).

During this initial visit, you will probably be asked to keep a "pain diary" for about four weeks. The diary should log every detail you can muster about your headaches—what seems to set them off, what has happened before they begin, how long they last, and what happens after they end, as well as describing the nature of the headache pain and any accompanying conditions.

At this point, many people become impatient. They want biofeedback to work as quickly as medication, to be the "fast, fast, fast relief" that television commercials promise for their products.

Of course, your headaches are painful and you want them to end as soon as possible. But draw on your reserves of patience. Biofeedback usually takes about four to six weeks to show results, as opposed to about two to four weeks for preventive medication, and ten to sixty minutes for symptomatic medication. On the other hand, the results you do eventually get from biofeedback will be all your doing, not a "quick fix" from a pill. It takes longer to learn biofeedback than it does to medicate yourself, but the results should last longer, and there will be no side effects.

Once you learn the technique of biofeedback, you can practice it for a lifetime.

THE TRAINING BEGINS

On your second visit, the biofeedback therapist will take you to a dimly lit, quiet room. You'll be given a comfortable chair and shown the equipment. The biofeedback therapist will show you the type of feedback that you will receive. This may be an oscillating tone, a beep that changes pitch, a meter, a digital readout, a flashing light, a column of lights, or, in some cases, the reaction of the therapist as he or she reads the machine.

THE SKILLS OF BIOFEEDBACK

Once you understand what the feedback will be, you can begin to learn how to get the response you want. Relaxing your muscles, or raising your hand temperature (which means that more blood is flowing into your hands, relieving the pressure on the blood vessels in your head) will lower a tone, or cause a light to stop flashing. When you get the result you want, you can monitor your body. How does your body feel when the machine says it's "relaxed"?

You can use this feedback to learn the following skills, which will likely be taught in the following order:

1. *Body awareness and breathing exercises.* As we've seen, being aware of your body is the first step to changing its responses. Simply being asked to focus on different parts of your body, especially those parts related to headache, or those parts where you tend to express your own tension, may be a revelation. Many people with headaches have developed a high pain threshold and the ability to be productive under almost any circumstance. These are admirable traits, but they may have been achieved by means of blocking out pain or awareness of bodily discomfort. Focusing on discomfort, with an eye toward correcting it, will not necessarily make you any less productive—and is the first step toward reducing your headache pain.

We deal with breathing exercises in more detail in Chapter 5. For now, let us just point out that deep breathing is essential both for relaxation and for providing adequate oxygen to the blood, which in turn helps the blood flow and feeds the tissues.

2. *Progressive relaxation and deep muscle exercise.* "Progressive relaxation" is a concept first developed by Dr. Edmund Jacobson in 1929. It refers to the process of "progressively" relaxing first one, then another, set of skeletal muscles.

At the same time that he described this technique, Dr. Jacobson also related its use in his successful treatment of four cases of muscle contraction headache. We now know that this technique can benefit migraineurs, as well.

We describe a progressive relaxation technique that you can use yourself in Chapter 5. Basically, it involves relaxing first your feet, then your calves, then your thighs, and so on, on through the muscles in your scalp.

"Deep muscle exercise" is a technique for first contracting, then relaxing, certain muscles. By focusing on contracting first, you're able to become aware of the muscle, and aware of your ability to affect it. Once you've contracted a muscle voluntarily, it becomes easier to relax it.

3. *Passive relaxation and guided imagery exercises.* Passive relaxation refers to a state of mind where you are no longer "trying" to do anything. You're not even trying to relax! Instead, you simply allow your attention to rest with your breathing or your body awareness, rather than striving to "pay attention" to anything in particular. Troubling or stimulating thoughts may cross your mind during passive relaxation, but rather than trying to address them, or to shut them out, you simply allow them to pass through and be forgotten.

Passive relaxation is the goal of many forms of meditation. Again, in Chapter 5 we go into more detail about how you can achieve this state on your own.

We also discuss guided imagery in Chapter 5. Basically, guided imagery is a process of imagining yourself in relaxing situations, such as lying on the beach or sitting in a warm, sunny field. With practice, simply calling up the image can trigger a relaxed response in your body.

4. *Scalp, facial, shoulder, and neck relaxation.* Now that you've learned how to relax, you can focus on specific body areas that are especially likely to be involved in your headaches. The specific feedback from the biofeedback machines will help to increase your awareness of these areas and their various states.

5. *Limb warmth and limb heaviness.* A body part feels warm and heavy because of the amount of blood that is flowing through it. As we've seen, variations in blood flow are often related to both migraine and muscle contraction headaches. In both types of headaches, an insufficient flow of blood to the brain before the headache seems to trigger an excess flow of blood to the head (temporal artery) during the headache. This accounts for the throbbing feeling that many migraineurs experience, as well as for the tightness experienced in a muscle contraction headache.

Therefore, if blood can be drawn away from the head and into the arms and legs, blood flow can be stabilized and the pressure and pain relieved. Getting your limbs to feel warm and heavy may mean that you are drawing more blood into your limbs and away from your head. Interestingly, you can get your limbs to feel warm—and therefore to be full of blood—simply by imagining them so. Learning how to make your imagination work for you in this way is part of this stage of biofeedback training.

6. *Autogenic, or self-directed phrases to induce relaxation.* "Autogenic" means self-generated. An autogenic phrase used in biofeedback training would be something like "I am very relaxed," or "My hands and feet are quite warm," or "I feel calm and peaceful."

You may be wondering what the purpose is of making these statements about yourself if you do not in fact feel that way. Particularly if you are experiencing a headache, or the stress that may contribute to one, you will not be feeling relaxed or peaceful, and your hands are likely to be quite cold from unstable blood flow to the brain. Why then make these statements?

The answer is, once again, because of the power of your mind—in this case, the power of suggestion. Researchers have found that simply making a statement about yourself may cause that statement to become true.

A dramatic example of the mind's power of suggestion comes from another field entirely. In a striking study, researchers gave some subjects alcoholic beverages while telling them that they had only received plain soda. They gave other subjects soda but told them that they had received alcohol. Large proportions of each group responded, not according to the physical properties of the drink they had imbibed, but according to what they had been told about it. In other words, the people who believed themselves to be getting drunk became drunk, even though they had received no physical stimulus to make them so. They staggered around the room, experienced dizziness, and seemed to lose control of various faculties. Many of the people who believed they were sober showed no such behavior, even though when they were given alcoholic beverages that were labeled as such, they did show signs of inebriation.

Of course, you can try these results on yourself in a much less dramatic way. Try telling yourself that you're anxious, or angry, or sad, and see how quickly you really become that way. Unfortunately, people are often far more willing to "talk themselves into" a bad mood than a good one!

By the way, in Chapter 5, we have a more detailed discussion on autogenic suggestion and its uses for relieving headaches and stress.

YOUR BIOLOGICAL RESPONSE

Overall, in biofeedback, you will be learning how to experience muscle relaxation throughout your head, neck, and body. The blood vessels in your hands and feet will dilate, or expand, leading to warmth in your fingers and toes. There may also be an increase in blood flow to some parts of the brain, along with a decreased blood flow through some of your scalp arteries, such as the temporal arteries, which may become swollen during a migraine.

These changes in blood flow are caused by a decrease in catecholamines, the neurotransmitter chemicals, such as noradrenaline, which are produced by your adrenal glands during the "fight or flight" response. Normally, when you're faced with stress, these catecholamines are secreted and circulated throughout your bloodstream. They stimulate the blood vessels to constrict—and in turn stimulate the production of prostaglandins, which cause other blood vessels to expand. Relaxation decreases the presence of catecholamines, which prevents the whole destabilizing process from starting in the first place.

In addition, you will experience a shift of blood flow from your large muscles to your digestive organs. (You can see that stress—the experience of danger—would cause exactly the opposite reaction. A body facing danger would need all its blood in its large muscles, so it could fight or run away.) There may be an increase in your stomach's motility, or ability to move. That is, rather than remaining rigid and contracted, as it does in stress, your stomach is also relaxed.

Likewise, there may be an increase in your salivation (as opposed to the "dry mouth" people sometimes notice when they are anxious or frightened). Your eyes may water, and you may notice a decrease in perspiration or sweaty palms (again, the opposite of a stress reaction). (For more about stress, see Chapter 5.)

FOLLOW-UP

Your biofeedback therapist will work with you throughout several sessions, teaching you the skills we have described. He or she may give you audio cassettes for home practice, with recorded relaxation exercises or guided imagery processes ("Imagine yourself on a warm, sunny beach. Hear the water. Feel the warm sun on your shoulders, your hands . . .").

You may also be asked to keep a debriefing log, to record your sensations after doing your home relaxation exercises. Remember that the goal of this training is greater awareness, which leads to greater ability to affect your body's processes. Keeping a log is one way to become more aware. You may also be asked to continue your headache log, similar to the one on page 271. This will give you a chance to become even more aware of what sets your headaches off and how you respond to them. The log is a useful tool for you and your therapist to figure out what's working about the training and what is not.

In later sessions, your therapist may give you home biofeedback monitors. These usually take the form of thermal rings, which measure heat in your hands. Heat is an indicator of blood flow, and thermal rings are especially useful to those who suffer from migraine headaches. Or you may be given a portable EMG, another type of biofeedback monitor used by those with muscle contraction headaches to measure the amount of muscle contraction in various muscles.

Finally, your therapist may give you mini-exercises to do throughout your day. For example, "clench your jaw; now relax your jaw," "tighten and relax your shoulders," or "close your eyes for three minutes and imagine yourself lying on a sandy beach with the sun beating down and the sound of the waves in the distance." Many people with headaches find these periodic check-ins quite helpful. You may also schedule "booster" sessions to review biofeedback training with your therapist after several months.

BIOFEEDBACK MACHINES

There are two main types of biofeedback machines currently in use. A third monitor is used mainly in research, but may soon be available for clinical practice.

ELECTROMYOGRAPHIC (EMG) FEEDBACK

This type of monitor has most often been used for people with muscle contraction headaches. The machine graphs electrical information about the functioning of various muscles that seem to be involved in these headaches.

If you are using one of these machines, the biofeedback therapist will first clean your forehead with alcohol, then attach three electrodes there. Usually you get one electrode on the frontalis muscle over each eye with a third ground electrode in between.

Sometimes other placements are used, either at first or

later in the treatment. If you think about the various places that tense up when your head hurts, you can imagine some of these locations. For example, the cheek area over the masseter muscle, which controls biting, is one common placement. That's because some people clench their teeth when they're tense. Likewise, electrodes may be placed above and slightly in front of your ear, in the hairline over the temporalis muscle, which controls the jaw.

A third common placement is the back of your neck or the shoulder area over the trapezius muscle. This is the muscle that runs directly under the skin from near the bottom of the skull to cross the shoulder and into the upper back (for further discussion of various muscles and their relationship to headache, see Chapter 5).

Once the electrodes are in place, the machine is turned on. They measure the electrical force that is generated during muscle tension. The electricity is measured in microvolts, or millionths of a volt. This extremely low electrical signal is amplified by the equipment, while other electrical signals in the vicinity are screened out. Electricity is running only from you to the machine, not the other way around!

With everything ready, you are asked to relax. The machine then measures the electrical force generated by the muscle tension in your forehead (or in whatever other place the electrodes are attached). That's your threshold—the level of relaxation that you are initially able to achieve.

The machine is set to produce a soft tone to correspond to this threshold. Then you are asked to "relax more." Decontracting your muscles even further, to achieve this greater relaxation, makes the tone stop.

When you are consistently able to achieve this new, deeper level of relaxation, the machine's threshold is reset accordingly. Then you are asked to "relax still more." Once again, deeper relaxation makes the tone cease.

The process continues until you have achieved full relaxation of the muscle involved. Then electrodes may be moved to your neck, shoulders, jaw, cheeks, temples, or ears, so that you have experienced full relaxation of those muscles as well.

Once you have experienced this relaxation, as monitored by the machine, you can use your relaxation techniques more effectively to recreate the experience.

THERMAL FEEDBACK

Another type of biofeedback monitors your finger temperature. Since increasing the blood flow to your hand raises the temperature there, monitoring temperature is another way of measuring the blood flow to your hand.

This type of feedback uses a thermistor, a device that transforms heat into electrical energy. Then the electricity can be measured. Usually the thermistor is attached to the pad of one finger, but it may be put on the back of one finger. Since one hand is usually warmer than the other, it's important to keep putting the thermistor in the same place. The thermistor is attached to your skin with porous paper tape that will not trap any heat between the tape and your skin.

As you relax, more blood flows into your hands, so their temperature increases. A pleasantly hot sensation would correspond to the mid-90-degree range Fahrenheit. (Since some heat is lost through the skin, your skin temperature will never be as high as the normal blood temperature of 98.6 degrees.) The low 90s would be experienced as warm, the mid-80s as cool, and below 80 degrees, down to the room temperature of 72 degrees, as cold.

Because blood flow is so often related to migraine, thermal feedback is often used for migraineurs.

EXTRACRANIAL BLOOD VOLUME PULSE FEEDBACK

This method isn't yet used clinically, but may soon offer help to those with migraines and other vascular headaches. It uses a photoplethysmograph, a photoelectric cell that transmits light to a diode that in turn emits light.

The photoplethysmograph monitors the light reflected by a small area of skin. The more opaque the skin is, the lower the intensity of light reflected from it. As the heart pumps more blood through an artery, the skin above the artery becomes more opaque. Thus, by measuring the amount of light reflected off the skin, the machine is measuring the different amounts of blood that flow from one pulse to the next.

The feedback display for this machine is a series of lights that reflect the relative amount of blood each heartbeat pushes through an artery. This allows migraineurs to experience the flow of blood through the extracranial temporal artery—the artery that runs along the outside of the skull in the temple in front of the ear. The site of migraine pain is usually the site that is measured in this process, since scientists hypothesize that to be the site of increased blood flow when the artery becomes distended.

BIOFEEDBACK: PREVENTING HEADACHES OR RELIEVING THEIR SYMPTOMS

One of the most exciting aspects of biofeedback techniques is their apparent ability both to prevent headaches and to relieve pain if headaches do occur. One study reveals that of 154 randomly selected headache patients who had used biofeedback up to four years earlier, a majority had experienced improvement in both areas. Some 69 percent of the 154 had had combined migraine and muscle contraction headaches before treatment, 67 percent had reported daily headache pain, and 33 percent had experienced constant pain.

The study showed that some 56 percent of those with combined headaches were still reporting at least 50 percent improvement. Of those who had completed treatment from two to four years later, 57 percent were also reporting at least 50 percent improvement in preventing and relieving headache.

Of these 154 patients, 95 percent reported that biofeedback had given them some ability to remain calm during the headache itself. About one-half had some success in stopping the headache completely, although only 8 percent with migraines and 15 percent with muscle contraction headaches could stop their headaches consistently.

Although complete freedom from pain during headache wasn't a result for most biofeedback clients, the overwhelming majority reported a variety of other benefits. For migraineurs and muscle contraction headache sufferers, 95 percent said that biofeedback had helped them to remain calm; 81 percent and 92 percent, respectively, said it had helped them to reduce the intensity of their headaches; 80 percent and 87 percent said that biofeedback had helped them to take less medication; 73 percent and 89 percent said it had reduced the time their headaches lasted; and 49 percent and 86 percent said that it enabled them to stop their headaches completely on some occasions.

As for preventing headaches, only about one-third of the migraineurs could prevent headaches triggered by food, weather, or menstrual cycles. Apparently, the most difficult type of migraine to control with biofeedback is the menstrual migraine (for more on this topic, see Chapter 8). However, some 80 percent of migraineurs and 84 percent of those with tension headaches said that biofeedback had helped them to prevent headaches that they identified as being triggered by stress. Interestingly, children who learn biofeedback are more likely to be able to prevent their headaches than adults who learn it.

MAXIMIZING THE EFFECTS OF BIOFEEDBACK

How can you tell whether biofeedback will be an effective technique for you? There are no hard and fast rules about who benefits from this method of learning relaxation. We have, however, made some observations and drawn some conclusions from the research published by others:

Biofeedback works best for those who achieve the greatest degree of physiological control. As you might expect, those who are most successful in achieving the physical goals of biofeedback are those who go on to be most successful in controlling their headaches. The studies we cited earlier suggest that the idea of "success" may be of equal or greater importance than any actual physical result. But it seems that migraineurs who can raise their finger temperatures to at least 95 degrees Fahrenheit (representing almost total blood vessel expansion) and muscle contraction headache people who can lower their forehead EMG rating to below one microvolt (representing almost total muscle relaxation) are most likely to show improvement.

However, it's important to note that in addition to the actual reduction of headache pain, people report other good benefits from biofeedback. A greater sense of relaxation, a heightened sense of power in coping with daily stress, and a generally more positive outlook on life are all results that people have reported from this treatment, regardless of its effect on their headaches.

Likewise, even some who have not achieved these physical results of temperature or voltage have nevertheless achieved great improvement in the treatment of their headaches.

Biofeedback works best for those who use relaxation techniques most frequently. People who use relaxation techniques daily—even for brief periods of time—are most likely to show the most improvement. In one study, some 69 percent of those showing an overall improvement of 50 percent or more were using relaxation techniques every day. Of those whose headache improvement was less than 50 percent, only 39 percent were using relaxation techniques every day.

Of those with 50 percent or more improvement, some 53 percent continued to practice a ten-minute or more extended period of relaxation at least once a week. Of those with less than 50 percent improvement, only 33 percent continued to practice an extended period of relaxation.

BIOFEEDBACK AND MEDICATION

What about those of you who are unwilling to give up your medication, even while you are eager to try something new that may someday replace it? Can biofeedback work for you?

The answer, depending on the type of medication you take, is probably yes. As we saw in Chapter 3, continued use of analgesics (pain relievers such as aspirin, Tylenol, Advil, or Nuprin) or of vasoconstrictors (ergotamine compounds, such as Cafergot) can cause a rebound effect, in which the headache becomes more severe and lasts longer, despite the medication. Eventually, someone suffering from analgesic or ergotamine rebound effect is taking daily overdoses of medication while still experiencing frequent or constant headache pain. For any treatment to work, including biofeedback, it's necessary to withdraw from the medication. However, your doctor or health care practitioner may suggest alternatives to help you through the withdrawal period.

Likewise, benzodiazepines (tranquilizers, such as Valium), should be discontinued for biofeedback to be effective. These medications tend to interfere with a person's awareness of his or her body, as well as to blunt the effects of stress. Since the goal of biofeedback is to increase physical and emotional awareness, taking tranquilizers puts you at cross purposes with pain management.

Other types of medication are effective when used with biofeedback. However, in one study of headache patients using biofeedback, 64 percent of those using preventive medication said that biofeedback had helped them to reduce headache pain. As many as 37 percent said that a combination of biofeedback and medication had led to the total elimination of their headaches.

What types of medication may be used with biofeedback? Apparently beta blockers like propranolol HCl (Inderal) or the antidepressants like amitriptyline HCl (Elavil or Endep) may be effective. Propranolol prevents blood vessel dilation and is also a serotonin antagonist, which means that it helps to stabilize blood flow. Thus it and biofeedback training are suited to work in tandem. However, studies have shown that beta blockers may affect people's ability to learn how to warm their hands through biofeedback. In addition, since depression may be a side effect of propranolol, persons taking this medication who do become depressed, may achieve fewer of biofeedback's beneficial side effects, notably its sense of increased power and control.

Amitriptyline HCl increases brain levels of serotonin, which also has a beneficial effect on the brain's perception of pain and tendency to depression. It is a tricyclic antidepressant, although for those who suffer from headaches without depression, its emotional effects will not be noticeable. Its chemical makeup is compatible with the goals of biofeedback, which may be used to reduce and eventually eliminate this medication altogether.

Ask your doctor about other preventive medications, and/or appropriate amounts of symptomatic medications that may be taken during biofeedback training.

BIOFEEDBACK AND ITS SIDE EFFECTS

We've talked a lot about the side effects of medication. But what about biofeedback? Doesn't it have any side effects?

Like any other treatment, biofeedback does have side effects. As we discussed in Chapter 3, "side" effects is really a misnomer. Because the human body is complex, and in a complex relationship with the human mind, *anything* we do is bound to have more than one effect. The good news about biofeedback is that most if *its* side effects are positive. And potential negative side effects are extremely rare.

The positive side effects in biofeedback include improved sleep patterns, an elevation in mood, and an increased sense of power and control in one's life. In one study of 154 patients who used biofeedback, some three out of four reported improvement in sleep and mood. In another study, migraineurs who successfully used temperature biofeedback showed positive changes in their scores on the MMPI (Minnesota Multiphasic Personality Inventory), a commonly used psychological test. Patients using propranolol (Inderal) who had successfully controlled their migraines showed no such improvements on the MMPI.

BIOFEEDBACK VS.
OTHER METHODS OF RELAXATION

Except for one study, there is little data that compares biofeedback with other headache treatments, owing to the lack of researchers' interest in nonmedical relaxation techniques. Fortunately, Dr. Blanchard and his colleagues did conduct a study that suggested that biofeedback can help those who are not helped by other relaxation techniques.

In this study, 78 percent of those with mixed headaches who had not been helped by progressive relaxation were helped by thermal biofeedback. And 43 percent of those with migraines who had not been helped by progressive relaxation showed a 50 percent or greater improvement after thermal biofeedback.

The results were similar for muscle contraction headaches. Some 47 percent of those who had not been helped by relaxation techniques found relief of at least 50 percent by using EMG biofeedback.

Dr. Blanchard's figures support the idea that biofeedback is a technique to be reckoned with, and certainly one that you should consider if you are dissatisfied with or apprehensive about other methods. While we believe the relaxation, meditation, and guided imagery techniques described in Chapter 5, as well as the exercise and massage described in Chapter 6, to be extremely helpful, some people are simply not comfortable with these methods. They may feel reassured by the scientific support for biofeedback, or by its greater similarity to other medical procedures. Some people also use biofeedback as a jumping-off point, a "first taste" of relaxation training that may later expand to include massage, meditation, and the other methods outlined in the next two chapters.

[5]

LETTING GO OF THE PAIN:
THERAPIES
AND RELAXATION TECHNIQUES

MIND AND BODY: A HOLISTIC APPROACH
TO YOUR HEADACHES

As WE SAY REPEATEDLY throughout this book, there is
rarely a single "cause" of your headaches. If you get recurrent, frequent headaches, you probably have a biological
tendency rooted in some chemical or neurological disorder
in the brain. This tendency, however, may be triggered by
psychological, dietary, or environmental factors, or by some
combination of the three.

In this chapter, we'll consider the psychological aspect
of headaches: what emotional factors may set them off, and
the ways in which we can enlist our mind in preventing or
reducing their pain.

Many people resist a psychological discussion of their
headaches. They feel that it trivializes the very real pain
they suffer, and ignores their sense of helplessness or frustration at the way headaches disrupt their lives. They may
feel that they're being told to "change their personalities,"
or get the message that if they would "just relax," they
could spare themselves unnecessary pain. Perhaps they secretly fear that their headaches *are* "their fault," or that this
syndrome indicates that "something is wrong" with them.

If any of these concerns are in your mind, we'd like to
set the record straight. Your headaches may indeed be a

message from yourself that something is not working as well as it could in your life. It may indeed be true that making a change in how you think about some aspect of your life, or in how you act, will go a long way toward alleviating your headaches. This is quite different from feeling that there is something wrong with you or that you need to make major alterations in your personality.

For many years, it was popular among doctors to attribute headaches to a "headache personality." People who got headaches were supposed to be tense and driven, have difficulty expressing their anger, have high standards for themselves and others, and be more than usually eager for the approval of others.

Now we know that there is no such thing as a headache personality. People of all different personalities get headaches, and many people with the so-called headache personality don't get headaches. However, it may be that personality traits such as the ones profiled above help trigger stress or aggravate behavior that leads to headaches. From that point of view, looking at psychological factors as well as all other factors only makes sense.

Some of the ideas we suggest in this chapter may not seem to fit you or your situation. Some may make you uncomfortable. Some may resonate with your ideas about yourself or seem to fit your situation. Whatever your response, we urge you to keep an open mind. Many people have headaches, and all of us have psychological patterns that sometimes help us, sometimes get in our way. If you can take an honest look at your own patterns, without blaming or judging yourself, you may be able to make some changes that will go a long way toward reducing your headache pain.

ASK YOURSELF . . .

Here are some questions that you might ask yourself to begin your exploration. Remember, there are no right or wrong answers to these questions. The purpose of asking them is to discover something new about yourself and your headaches. If you find a particular idea just doesn't seem right to you, you'll probably let it pass by. But if a particular idea makes you angry, upsets you, or leads you to have long mental arguments about it, we may have hit a responsive chord. Allow yourself to have your reactions, keeping in mind that the more you learn about yourself, the more tools you'll have for restructuring the patterns that lead to your headaches.

- Do you believe that since one or both of your parents have headaches, you are "doomed" to have them, too? Do you think that you don't deserve a better fate than theirs?
- Do you believe that headaches are completely out of your control?
- Do you experience your headaches as a punishment for something you've done wrong?
- Do you think that your headaches are "your fault," because you live a stressful life, or don't handle stress well?
- Do you think your body is a hostile force that's somehow "out to get you"?
- Is it hard for you to say you're angry with someone, especially someone you love?
- Is it hard for you to say no, or to admit that you don't have the time or energy to do something you'd like to do?
- Have you ever found that having a headache meant that you didn't have to do something that you kind of wished you could get out of anyway?
- Do you sometimes wish someone would take care of *you*, instead of you always being the one to take care of everyone?
- Do you wake up looking forward to your days, or do you frequently wake up with a feeling of dread, fear, or frustration?
- Do you love yourself? Do you like yourself?
- When was the first headache you remember having? What were you doing? How were you feeling?

What are the first thoughts that come to mind now that you've read through this list of questions? How are you feeling? Run a quick check on your body. Are you feeling tension anywhere? Where? Are there other times when you feel this way?

Answering these questions may lead you to some insights about yourself and your headaches. You may find that some of your thoughts are illogical, or that your feelings don't seem to make sense. That doesn't matter. Many of our thoughts and feelings don't have logical explanations, but they may nevertheless be powerful influences in our lives. Remember: You're not alone. All human beings have painful and uncomfortable feelings, and all of us have limits. This will always be true, but becoming aware is the first step toward making changes.

STRESS IN OUR LIVES

Before we go on to discuss relaxation techniques, however, let us say a few words about stress. Many of us tend to think of stress as a bad thing. We may have the idea that we should be able to handle any type of stress with total calm, and to feel inadequate if we cannot.

Neither of these thoughts is accurate. From a scientific point of view, stress is any demand placed by the environment or by the body itself on the body. If you go out into a cold snowstorm, your body experiences thermal stress, and it mobilizes its forces to get warm. If you fall madly in love and your beloved says that he or she shares your feelings, the elation that you feel is also experienced as stress.

Thus the goal of relaxation techniques and other therapies is not to eliminate stress from our lives. As scientists who work in the field of stress are fond of saying, you can only eliminate stress totally by being dead. A life without responsibility, excitement, challenges, or strong emotion would certainly be very like a living death.

It's true that feeling anger, responsibility, or concern may also be stressors (causes of stress) upon our system. And if we feel that we shouldn't express our anger (say, at our children, or at our boss); can't handle our responsibility; or can't do anything about our concern, the level of stress increases. Thus the goal of the techniques in this chapter is to change the way we cope with stress.

No living human being with an active life can or should try to avoid all stress—or all discomfort. But the discomfort of headache pain *can* be avoided, at least to a great extent.

THE BIOLOGICAL BASIS OF STRESS

Dr. Hans Selye, the pioneer of stress study, has identified two types of stress. *Local adaptation syndrome* is the stress of your body trying to respond to a very specific (or local) stressor. For example, if you walk into a cold snowstorm, your body increases its metabolism, trying to warm you up. Usually, local adaptation matches the stressor, causing few health problems.

However, the *general adaptation syndrome* is the type of body reaction in which the defense may cause more problems than the threat. This syndrome is also known as the "fight or flight" response, because your body is reacting as though it had either to fight or to run for its life.

If the stressor you were facing were a wild bear in the woods, this might be a helpful reaction. But if the stressor is a fight with your boss—or the memory of a fight with your boss—your body's mobilization is excessive for the task at hand.

What happens in this reaction? Your pituitary gland may be stimulated to produce certain hormones that in turn stimulate the pancreas to secrete insulin. The insulin enables you to metabolize your blood sugar, so that your body can use it for energy.

For those of you with hypoglycemia, however, this may set off a chain reaction that leads to a headache, as well as to the other symptoms of hypoglycemia: confusion, irritability, loss of concentration, anxiety, depression, and sometimes uncontrollable crying or fits of temper (for more details, see Chapter 7). These reactions only increase your body's sense of danger and thus increase your stress.

Even for those of you without hypoglycemia, your body's mobilization may cause muscles to contract or blood vessels to constrict, setting off a muscle contraction, migraine, or mixed headache. However, if you can learn either to react differently to the stressor, or to relax your muscles and blood vessels after your initial stressed reaction, you can do a great deal to prevent or reduce your headaches.

RELAXATION TECHNIQUES

DEEP RELAXATION

Dr. Herbert Benson, a Harvard cardiologist, has discovered that when the human body is in a state of deep relaxation, many beneficial effects result. One is that the sympathetic nervous system slows down. The sympathetic nervous system is one-half of the autonomic nervous system—the functions of our body that happen "automatically," without our thinking about them. Specifically, the functions of the sympathetic nervous system include regulating the size of our pupils, the rate of our heartbeats, the size of our blood vessels, the level of our blood pressure, and the production of sweat. The sympathetic nervous system also regulates sleep, as well as feelings of alertness and relaxation. You can see why slowing this system down would lead to feeling relaxed while altering many of the physical conditions that lead to headaches.

Other beneficial physical changes occur during deep relaxation. The relaxed person takes fewer breaths per minute, yet breathes more deeply, "bathing" the blood cells in a refreshing bath of oxygen. More blood reaches the brain, which seems to help prevent headache.

In addition, the state of relaxation produces a lower level of *catecholamines*, which are the neurotransmitters (chemicals that transmit messages within the brain) that seem to stimulate headache in some people. Noradrenaline is one catecholamine that seems to be involved in headaches.

Further, during relaxation, the brain waves become less random and more synchronized. They also become closer to the *alpha state*, which is the name scientists have for the pattern of electrical activity in the brain that corresponds to the state of being relaxed and awake.

Since the brain controls body function, these latter two responses produce beneficial effects throughout the body. In fact, in this state, the body begins to heal itself, repairing many of the strains brought about by the daily wear and tear of stress.

Interestingly, the stress reaction is automatic, but the relaxation response is not. However, it can be learned. And when you master the relaxation technique that is right for you, you can practice it or some version of it at any time or place, even in the midst of a stressful, demanding day.

DEEP BREATHING

Dancers, actors, and other performers know firsthand the relaxing effects of deep breathing. They use it to combat stage fright—an exciting but sometimes paralyzing form of stress! If you learn deep breathing techniques, you can "bring yourself down" into a state of calm, relaxed concentration whenever you take the time to do so.

First, practice breathing through your nose. The nose is lined with little hairs called *cilia,* which clean impurities and pollutants out of the air. Thus your brain gets cleaner air through the nose. The air also seems to go more directly into your brain when you breathe through your nose. Try breathing first through your mouth, then through your nose —you'll feel the difference right away!

Then, learn how to breathe all the way down into your diaphragm (the area just below your abdomen, more or less where your stomach is). When you inhale, you should feel yourself filling up with air. Your stomach should puff out slightly, your rib cage and lungs should feel full, and the air should penetrate well below your chest.

The easiest way to feel diaphragm breathing is to lie flat on your back, either on a firm mattress or on the floor. Place your hand lightly on your stomach and take a deep breath in. Feel how the air just falls into your body, filling you and pushing out your stomach; then feel the sense of collapse as you let the air float out. Think of the air as "falling" and "floating," so that your breathing isn't work, but a response to a natural inner impulse.

When you can sense what deep breathing feels like,

slow your breathing down. Breathe in to a slow count of four, hold the breath for four counts, then breathe out to a slow count of four. When you have mastered this, breathe in and out on a count of eight, holding the breath for four in between. Continue to expand the amount of time your inhaling and exhaling takes, paying particular attention to keeping your exhaling slow and even.

Once you have mastered the rhythm of deep breathing, you may wish to imagine yourself breathing in relaxation, calm, comfort, love, or some other healing image, while breathing out tension, worry, fear, or whatever is causing your stress.

A breathing technique that is especially useful when you are hurrying to get somewhere in a car or on public transportation is to slow your breathing down. Since you can't physically hurry, why not take the chance to relax, even if you are late? Breathe in on a count of one, and out on a count of one. Then up the count to two, then three, and so on, until you feel your breaths are as long and slow as they can be, up to about twelve counts.

Some doctors feel that five minutes' worth of deep breathing is worth an hour's nap in terms of feeling refreshed and relaxed. The oxygen you take in both relaxes and energizes your brain cells, "erasing" the stressful effects that have come before.

You can also try deep breathing when you are about to get a headache, or even after you are in the throes of one. Concentrating on the breathing has a calming influence that takes your mind off the pain, and the physical effects of the breathing may serve to relieve some or all of the discomfort.

Many people discover, when they come to try deep breathing, that they are quite resistant to "slowing themselves down" in this way. The rhythm of frenetic work may be so compelling that it becomes difficult to take a five-minute time out to relax, even if one is far more efficient as a result. If you notice this resistance in yourself, acknowledge it, and be aware of how acting on it may contribute to your headaches. Perhaps you could try a time-limited experiment of a week in which you commit yourself to two relaxation breaks a day, then reconsider the process at the end of the week. Of course, once you've learned the technique of deep breathing, you can do it sitting up, even at your office desk!

PROGRESSIVE RELAXATION

Unlike the breathing techniques, which can be practiced at any time, this technique should first be tried when your head is clear. Its purpose is to help you to become aware of what it feels like to be completely relaxed, so that you can recover that feeling as you become tense. Lie down on your back, on a good, firm mattress, or on a comfortable floor. You can put a pillow under your head, and/or under your knees if it makes you more comfortable.

Allow your breathing to become deep and even. Then inhale, hold your breath, and stiffen one arm while lifting it. Clench it as tightly as you can, contracting the muscles. When you are ready, exhale, slowly, while relaxing the arm and letting it drop. Repeat this process with the other arm; with each leg (pointing your toe as you raise the leg); with your abdomen (tighten it and lift it from the floor); with your shoulders and upper back (tensing up off the floor, to look at your toes); and with your face (contorting it tightly). Then say to yourself, "I am completely relaxed, and I feel wonderful." Allow yourself to remember the feeling, and to recall it at other moments so that you can bring it into your life.

OVERALL BODY RELAXATION

This is a similar exercise, but one that can be done even while you are having a headache. It takes about ten minutes altogether, and it should be done in privacy, somewhere you can lie down. Some people do it when they get home at the end of their workday, to relieve the built-up stresses of the day. Again, if you are worried about being busy, think of how much more available you will be to your family and yourself if you take these ten minutes for yourself.

Lie down, in the type of comfortable position we've described elsewhere. It helps to dim the lights and loosen your clothes. Begin the deep breathing you've learned, and continue it throughout the exercise.

The purpose of this exercise is to work your way through every part of your body, relaxing it. Begin with your toes, then your heels, then your ankles, calves, thighs, buttocks. Relax your abdomen and chest. Relax the muscles around the base of your spine, then in the middle of your back, then your upper back, then your shoulders. Work your way down your arms, to your elbows, your hands, your fingers. Work your way back up your arms, relaxing your shoulders again, then your neck, then your chin, your face, your eyes, your forehead.

Linger on each part of your body. If you feel tension, tell it to go away. Sometimes it helps to imagine puffing the tension away with each exhaled breath.

When you are completely relaxed, say to yourself, "It's safe to let go. It's safe to let go." Enjoy the feeling of being relaxed for a moment. Then stretch, and sit up very slowly. Allow the relaxed feeling to remain within you, or around you, as you move back into your activities.

Sometimes people will feel so relaxed that they fall asleep, possibly sleeping through a headache. Eventually, however, they come to associate relaxation with alertness as well as with sleep.

Some people like to do this exercise to a relaxation tape, which they or a friend records. Be sure the person speaking pauses about five or ten seconds between mention of each body part.

GUIDED RELAXATION AND CREATIVE VISUALIZATION
Other tapes are available for relaxation and visualization exercises (exercises in which you visualize images or situations that help you to relax). You may wish to buy one from your health food store or "New Age" bookstore.

RELAXATION BY THE NUMBERS
Here's a variation on the relaxation exercises that can be done sitting upright in a chair. Visualize a comfortable place, either real or imaginary—one in which you feel com-

pletely safe. Begin your deep breathing, allowing it to continue throughout the exercise.

When you have pictured the comfortable place in enough detail that you feel comfortable and safe, see a very large number three, then a medium-sized three, then a very small three. Repeat this process with the numbers two and one. Then say to yourself, "I am now relaxed and calm. My head is cool. My neck is cool. The rest of my body is warm and heavy. Now I am going to relax more deeply."

In order to relax more deeply, take a deep breath, hold it while counting down from ten to one, then exhale. You are now in deep relaxation, or the alpha state we described earlier, the condition of being relaxed yet awake. You might think of this state as the one your brain is in when you first wake up in the morning or are just about to drift off at night.

In this state, your mind is quite receptive. Use it to make some of the *autogenic* (self-generated) suggestions or affirmations that we discuss in the following section. You can plant suggestions in your mind that will help you to reduce and prevent your headaches as well as to enhance your self-confidence, self-image, and self-esteem.

ENLISTING THE AID OF YOUR MIND

The following techniques are based on the assumption that your mind can be a powerful ally in reducing and preventing your headache pain. You can use your mind's ability to create images, to analyze and explore, and to set up a general direction for your thinking. These abilities can open up new possibilities for healing yourself.

AUTOGENIC TRAINING.

This training is a type of self-hypnosis. In a sense, you "talk yourself into" a relaxed and positive state. The goal is for your body to feel warm (which means that your blood vessels are fully dilated, counteracting the constrictive phase of migraines) and heavy (which means that your muscles are fully relaxed, counteracting muscle contraction headaches).

The first few times you do this exercise, you'll probably want to do it lying down. Later, however, you can do it sitting up, which makes it another "portable" exercise.

Find a room that is dimly lit and well ventilated, where you can be sure of not being disturbed. Take off any jewelry or glasses you have on and loosen your clothes. Lie on a firm, comfortable surface, with or without pillows. (You might try placing a pillow below your knees if that makes it easier to relax your legs.) Lie with your legs slightly apart and your arms away from your body, so that you can experience each limb separately. Let yourself relax and go limp.

Begin your deep breathing. Then, when you are ready, begin to make some suggestions to yourself. Think these suggestions in the present tense, and in a positive mode. For example, "My right arm is warm and heavy. My left arm is warm and heavy. My right leg is warm and heavy. My left leg is warm and heavy." Continue on through your abdomen, chest, back, and shoulders. Tell yourself that your heartbeat is slow and powerful, and that your breathing is deep and relaxed. Tell yourself that your neck, and then your head, are heavy and cool (since the goal is to prevent excess blood—which causes both heat and headache—in your head).

Be sure your suggestions are all in this positive mode. If you say, "My arm is not tense," or "I'm not going to get a headache," the words "tense" and "headache" will ring far louder in your subconscious than the "nots" that precede them. Focus on how you want your body to feel by saying that it already feels that way.

At the end of the exercise, say to yourself, "I feel completely relaxed and refreshed." Pause, enjoy that feeling, then stretch and get up slowly.

Some people object to this technique, saying, "But I *don't* feel relaxed, so why should I say I am?" Scientific study has shown that this technique is based on the power of suggestion, which, as we know from the placebo effect, can be very powerful indeed. Try to suspend your disbelief for six or seven tries with this technique—every day for a week. If by that time, it doesn't work for you, you can always try something else.

While you are using this technique, be sure to pause between each suggestion, and to make each suggestion two times or however long is necessary until you feel what you are saying. If necessary, move on to another part of your body and return to the tense part later. You may not achieve total relaxation the first time, but with practice, this may be an effective technique for you.

CREATIVE IMAGERY

This technique can be used after a relaxation exercise, as the mind is most receptive to it when the body is fully relaxed. However, this is also a good method to use while you are having a headache. It's both a way of easing the headache pain and of learning something about the headache.

Find a relaxed position, possibly after five or ten minutes of doing a deep relaxation exercise to "bring yourself down." In any case, be sure you are doing deep, relaxed breathing. The focus on deep breathing allows you to clear your mind.

Then allow your mind's power to make images come to your aid. Use any one of the following images to ease either your tension or your headache pain. Don't use more than one at a time, but do experiment, trying out these images or ones you create yourself, until you find the ones that work for you.

See yourself lying in a cool stream, and imagine the water is washing away your headache, or your tension. See yourself wandering down a shady path in the woods and meeting a person whom you immediately trust and love, whether someone in your life or an imaginary person; that figure gives you a magic potion, which cures your headache as you drink it. See yourself gradually surrounded by a pure white light, which makes you feel very safe; as the white light flows through you, your headache lifts and dissolves. Picture a light that grows until it is a bright, pulsating mass; then it shrinks and disappears; then picture the same thing happening to your headache. Picture breathing your headache out into a cloud with every breath; imagine the cloud in detail, including its color, texture, and smell; then imag-

ine changing the cloud into a beautiful scene or object;
then imagine breathing that peaceful scene back into your
head.

A related technique is to allow an image of your headache to emerge. Perhaps you see it as a murky shape, or a
blazing fire, or as an animal with its claws in your head, or
as a bolt of lightning that attacks you. Allow the image to
emerge in as much detail as you can summon. Ask yourself
what color your headache is, how large it is, what its texture
is, what it smells like, whether it's making any noise. Allow
yourself simply to observe and study this image, without
either attraction or disgust, without thinking about what it
means or what it's saying about you.

Then, when you have a clear image in your mind, allow
yourself to change it. Some people find it helpful to ask the
image for permission to change it. If the headache is sharp,
imagine yourself gently buffing the pointy edges to make
them round. If your headache is a hot red, picture it slowly
changing to a cool blue. If your headache is an angry animal, picture yourself feeding and stroking the animal,
which gradually becomes tame and loving. Continue to
look for sensory details of sight, taste, smell, touch, and
sound, to allow the image to be as vivid as possible.

When you have created a particular image, you may
wish to keep it with you, or you may wish to picture send-
ing it on its way. When you feel complete, return to an
awareness of your body. Run through the various parts of
your body and tell any remaining tension to go away, continuing to breathe deeply. Stretch, and get up slowly.

An alternate use of this technique is to begin to ask
your headache questions after you have imaged it. Ask it
why it's here, what it's telling you, what it wants. Ask it
what you need to do to ease the pain and what you need to
do to prevent the pain. Allow your mind to wander freely
through these questions and answers. Try not to judge or
even think about the answers, phrases, images, or insights
that may float to the surface, even if they seem impossible
or don't fit in with your image of yourself. Allow yourself to
notice and remember them. When your conversation is
over, tell your headache that you've heard what it said and

respectfully ask it to leave. Return to your body and allow yourself to relax once again. Then stretch and sit up slowly.

After you've completed that exercise, you may find it helpful to write down your thoughts and feelings. Certainly it will be useful to jot down what your headache "told" you. You might then go on to allow your mind to wander through various thoughts and feelings that you have about the experience. If you pictured violent things happening to someone you know, this doesn't mean that you literally wish these things, but it may mean that you are angry and that your headache has been the place where your anger has been expressed. Possibly you can find another way to express that feeling, one that is not so hurtful to yourself. If you pictured wanting total escape from everyone in your life, this doesn't necessarily mean that you want such isolation, but it may mean that you are feeling burdened by others' needs and expectations and your headache has been your way of escaping from them. Perhaps you could deal with these feelings in another way. Many people find it useful to work through these changes with the help of a counselor or therapist, which we'll discuss in more detail in the next section.

Finally, one other useful imaging technique is to imagine yourself in a real-life situation that you find difficult or stressful, such as hurrying to meet a deadline, being yelled at by a boss, or being tempted by a food that you know will trigger a headache. Picture the situation in as much detail as you can, then imagine yourself responding to it differently: You relax and take some time out to organize your work and care for yourself; you yell back at your boss or calmly explain why she or he shouldn't treat you that way; you turn from the food to some other treat that brings you pleasure. Of course, you can use this technique even when you don't have a headache!

In addition to its curative powers, creative imagery can be an excellent way for you to learn more about what is bothering you or how you can find a creative solution to a problem. The trick is to allow yourself to image freely, without judging or drawing conclusions that might limit your imagination. Then, afterwards, allow any thoughts or feelings that you may have to come up. If you find yourself imagining disturbing images, you might change them to positive images during this process. Even if you don't "understand" what the images "mean," this can be a powerful healing tool.

USE OF COLOR IMAGERY

A variation on creative imagery is to imagine a healing color. Some people find the image of white light comforting. Others find that a cool blue is refreshing, or that a natural green brings a sense of peace. Picture yourself surrounded by a cloud of this color. Then, with every inhalation, breathe the color inside you. With every exhalation, breathe out to make room for more of the color. Continue to do your deep breathing, filling yourself with the healing color, for about five or ten minutes.

AFFIRMATIONS

These are similar to autogenic suggestions, but may be done in any state. They'll have the most impact if you do them just after you wake up, just before you fall asleep, or at another highly relaxed time during the day. However, you may also discover that saying them at times of tension has a calming influence. It's always helpful to combine any repeating of affirmations with a few moments of deep breathing.

Affirmations are positive statements about who you are and how you feel. Some affirmations that people find helpful are: I am calm and relaxed and I have time for everything I want to do; I love myself and I am loved by the people in my life; I am a valuable person who contributes a great deal to the people in my life; and so on. As with autogenic suggestions, affirmations should be in the positive mode: Saying "I'm not a bad person" will make you feel terrible!

You can say affirmations out loud, sing them to yourself, whisper them, or just think them in your mind. Some people find it helpful to write them down as a way of repeating them. Others like to carry written affirmations with them and read them at stressful moments. Many people are skeptical about the value in doing this, but discover un-imagined benefits when they actually give it a try.

You might want to focus on two or three affirmations a week, possibly changing them from week to week. Some people find it useful to post their affirmations where they can easily be seen—or where they will be seen at tense moments, such as by the phone, on the visor above the windshield, or in the bathroom.

A variation on the affirmations is positive reinforce-ment. Animal trainers find that rewarding an animal every time it does something right or even partly right is far more effective than punishing it when it does something wrong. Sports enthusiasts have also discovered that praising them-selves each time they do something well—or praising themselves for the effort they are making, regardless of its results—actually leads to startling improvements in their game.

Just as an experiment, you might try to focus on prais-ing yourself frequently, almost continually. Tell yourself, "Good for you, you're really a good person," or "Look at how much work you got done this morning." Even if you believe that you could have gotten more work done, focus on praising yourself for what you did do. If you want to start making negative judgments, tell yourself, "I can go back to that next week. This week I'm trying an experiment." As with affirmations and autogenic suggestions, you may find that "thinking positive" actually produces surprisingly good results—maybe even better than you hoped for while you were being self-critical!

MEDITATION

Various techniques in Yoga and Zen Buddhism involve meditation, which may be practiced in many different ways. The form known as Transcendental Meditation, or TM, has become popular in the West. It involves focusing on a mantra, or a single word. Practitioners of TM believe that you must be assigned your mantra, but you may also use *Om*, which means "whole," or if you prefer using a word in English, *one*.

The purpose of the mantra is to allow your mind to be

free of all its usual worries and concerns, by focusing only on the mantra. Find a comfortable place to sit, with your spine straight and your hands in your lap. Close your eyes and breathe deeply. Repeat your mantra each time you exhale, either silently or aloud. If other thoughts appear in your mind, allow them to pass through, without either focusing on them or resisting them. You can eventually work up to meditating ten to twenty minutes per day, one to three times a day. This "clearing" seems useful to many people.

THERAPY AND YOUR HEADACHES

Along with all the other physical and psychological approaches we've suggested, many people find it helpful to work with a psychotherapist. A therapist is trained at understanding human behavior. Time with a therapist is a chance for you to focus on yourself and your needs, and to discover some possibilities for fulfilling yourself and meeting some needs that you may have been ignoring or pushing away.

There are various types of therapists and various schools of therapy. Psychiatrists have degrees in medicine. Because of their long years in training, they tend to be the most expensive therapists. Some therapists have doctoral degrees in social work, psychology, or some related field. Other therapists have master's degrees in social work, psychology, or education. In addition to a master's degree, a therapist may be licensed, which represents a higher degree of accomplishment; or certified, which represents a still higher level. Fees may vary accordingly. However, many therapists offer a sliding scale or work at clinics where counseling is available at lower rates.

Discussing all the various schools of psychotherapy is beyond the scope of this book. We'd like to focus on two that have particular relevance for the treatment of headaches. However, we stress that neither of these schools may be the one that is best for you. If you find a therapist with whom you are compatible and whose approach appeals to you, working with that person will be beneficial, and will ultimately make a difference in your experience of headaches.

GESTALT

Gestalt therapy is based on the idea of the *gestalt*, or whole: the emotions, the thoughts, and the body. Gestalt therapists believe in helping clients to act out the various forces going on within them. For example, a gestalt therapist might hand a client a pillow and say, "Give your headaches to this pillow." The thoughts and feelings that come up as the client pummels the pillow would then be material for analysis; in addition, the very experience of "giving the headache away" might be helpful.

A gestalt therapist might work with a client on what the experience of a headache is like, and might help the client focus on experiencing the pain rather than fighting it. Many people find enormous relief in a therapy that focuses on their experience, particularly if they feel that elsewhere in their lives they are asked to suppress their own experience to focus on others'.

COGNITIVE/BEHAVIORAL THERAPY

This type of therapy has proved quite helpful to many people with chronic headaches. It's a combination of two therapeutic schools: cognitive and behavioral.

Cognitive therapy is based on the idea that many of our difficulties come from the way we think about things. If we can reshape our thoughts, we can reshape our experiences and our actions. For example, a negative thought such as "I never finish all the work I want to" might create stress and help trigger a headache. Changing that thought to "I've accomplished quite a lot and it's always possible to continue tomorrow" might be beneficial.

Behavioral therapy is based on the idea that it's possible to make small, concrete changes in our behavior that have powerful effects on our lives, even if we don't "understand" all the reasons why we previously acted the way we did. A cognitive/behavioral approach to therapy focuses on changing the thoughts and behaviors that may trigger headaches.

This approach often begins by asking the person who gets headaches to write down everything that happened before the headache, and everything that happened as a result of the headache. Note that the person is not trying to analyze causes or motivations, only to say what happened when.

For example, a person might write, "Before my headache, I got a call from our neighborhood bake sale and promised to bring some cookies tomorrow. I drove to school to pick the kids up. My husband called and said he'd be home from work late. When I was having my headache, I got another call from our local church, asking me to bring in some old clothes for their rummage sale. I was sick and upset, and told them I didn't have time to talk to them. I called my husband and told him I was sick, and he came home and watched the kids."

It's possible to imagine from this account that the person having the headache had difficulty saying no to requests, but that when she had a headache, she felt less uncomfortable about saying no. Similarly, she may have had difficulty asking her husband directly to share child care responsibilities, but having a headache allowed her to ask for his participation, or possibly to be offered his participation without her even having to ask. After all, she had a headache!

Of course, the woman in this example certainly wasn't having a headache "on purpose," in the sense that she had consciously planned to put herself in pain. But by identifying the possible "rewards" that accompanied her headache pain, a therapist could help her to get those rewards in another way. Possibly this would help reduce the headaches.

In addition, many people with headaches have negative reactions to the pain itself. They often feel angry, guilty, depressed, frustrated, or helpless as a result of having frequent headaches. Then they get upset about being upset! This vicious cycle of negative thoughts only increases the stress—and the pain.

Cognitive/behavioral therapy would focus on changing the negative thoughts to positive ones. Instead of thinking, "I'm such a failure; I can't even control my own life to prevent these headaches," the patient would be encouraged to think, "I'm doing a lot to cure myself, and I'm making a good start." Instead of thinking, "I can't control my headaches," the patient might think, "Trying to control my headaches doesn't seem to help; let me focus on experiencing them, instead." The patient might replace "What did I do wrong to cause this?" with "I wonder what I can learn from this experience."

Patients are often skeptical that these changes will help. However, even without a wholehearted belief in this technique, patients have been amazed at how much of a difference this "positive thinking" can make. Work with a therapist can help uncover places where thinking is negative and discover effective suggestions for positive thoughts to replace the self-blaming ones.

If you are willing to experiment, you might try making a list of your negative thoughts about your headaches, and then writing a list of corresponding positive thoughts. Carry the positive list—*without* the negative one!—and read it over when you are having a headache or feel you are about to have one. It may take a lot of repeating—after all, you've been repeating those negative thoughts for a long time, now—but you too may be surprised at the difference it makes.

HEADACHE PATTERNS AND SECONDARY GAINS

In the example we discussed above, a woman suffered a great deal from headache pain, but she also derived some benefits from her headaches. Therapists call these benefits "secondary gains"—the rewards we get from our suffering or our frustrations.

Many people find it difficult to accept the idea of secondary gains. They find it upsetting to imagine that they are in any way benefiting from an experience as painful and disrupting as a headache, or that they might be in any way reluctant to stop having headaches.

However, the positive side of this view is that it gives you a great deal more power over the events in your life. If you are in any way contributing to your headaches, that means you can act with equal effectiveness to prevent them, simply by changing your behavior. And it's important to remember that we don't cause ourselves pain because we enjoy pain, but because we may have learned we can't get the results we want in any other way. Perhaps sometimes there *is* no other way. But wouldn't you be willing to explore the possibility that there is, if it would help you to stop having headaches?

To this end, we list some of the typical secondary gains that people get from having headaches. If any of these results seem to match your experience with your headaches, we would counsel against blaming yourself or feeling guilty. Rather, we'd encourage you to think about what other ways you could accomplish the same ends. Again, a therapist can be a useful partner in that enterprise.

HEADACHES FOR ANGER

Sometimes, when we're angry with people we love, it's frightening to tell them so. We fear that they'll love us less, or maybe even leave us. At the very least, they may see that we're not the perfect person we wish we were; we're only human—we get angry.

If the people around you respond to your headaches with apologies, concern, and special treatment, you might consider whether this response is part of your "reward" for being sick. If the people around you respond to your headaches with anger of their own, this may also be a sign that they are responding to your anger.

HEADACHES FOR NURTURANCE

On the other hand, some of us feel that unless we are sick or needy, no one will take care of us or pay attention to us. We may have grown up in families where we only got loving treatment when we were sick, or where being sick was the one time we got special attention from our parents. These powerful psychological feelings like anger or powerful needs like nurturance, if not directly expressed, can drive the body to translate these emotions into physical pain.

If you find yourself expecting special treatment when you have a headache, you might consider whether there's some other way of getting that special treatment. Perhaps your family needs to establish a special day for each of its members, once a month, on which people are pampered and babied a little even when they are well.

BARRELING ON THROUGH

Some people take pride in not changing any aspect of their lives, even when they are nearly incapacitated from headache pain. They see their headaches as a personal challenge to which they will not succumb. If this profile fits you, you might consider what benefits you're getting from this behavior. Do you feel you then have the right to expect that other people will likewise have no limits or weaknesses when it comes to their obligations toward *you?* Do you feel that your endurance of pain and your sacrifices give you special rights in other areas? Do you feel secretly superior for being so strong? Or, on the other hand, are you afraid that *any* sign of weakness may reveal that you're really not as capable as you "should" be?

Again, the clue is to identify what you may be seeking —reassurance of your abilities, trust in others' ability to come through for you—and then to pursue that goal by other means than having a headache. The advantage of this way of thinking is that, even if psychological factors have nothing to do with your headaches, you've still learned something about yourself and found a new way to meet more of your needs.

WORKING TO OUR OWN ADVANTAGE

One final word of warning: Even if secondary gains are involved in our headache patterns, they aren't necessarily working to our advantage. Our coworkers' frustration with our absenteeism, or our family members' frustration with our frequent demands for quiet, may actually be preventing satisfying relationships at work or at home. This in turn raises our level of stress, creating the "need" for more headaches.

However, we may continue in our old patterns, simply because we don't believe that new ones are possible. The people around us may also be encouraging us to remain in those patterns, even if they are also frustrated with them. Our families may be annoyed—but continue to pamper us when we have a headache and at no other time. Our bosses may be irked, but still refuse to be reasonable in their expectations of us.

Changing old patterns may be hard. You can take comfort in knowing that everyone has these patterns, whether they work to change them or have adapted to them. The choice to face your patterns and struggle to change them may at first bring some discomfort, or even pain. But ultimately, the payoff in greater satisfaction can be worth a great deal.

[6]

GETTING PHYSICAL:
EXERCISE AND EXERCISES

IN ADDITION TO the psychological and mental approaches detailed in the previous chapter, there are many physical ways to prevent and relieve headaches. In Chapter 7, we'll talk about preventing headaches through diet. In this chapter, we'll talk about how exercise, massage, acupressure, and heat and cold can be used to reduce or hold off headache pain, and to reduce the frequency of your headaches.

WHEN YOU MUST RELIEVE A HEADACHE

Most of this chapter will be concerned with exercises that you can use to keep from having a headache. If you do get one, however, there are some drugless ways of bringing yourself some relief.

BREATHING
Whether you go on to focus on a physical exercise or a mental one, your deep breathing is one key to success. It will enable you to focus your mind on something other than your pain, while helping your body to relax, improving circulation, and bringing more oxygen into your bloodstream for a refreshing and energizing effect. To review the

fundamentals of deep breathing, see pages 151–53 in Chapter 5.

HEAT OR COLD?

Usually the rule is to apply heat before getting a headache, and to use ice when you are just starting to get one, or are in the throes of the headache itself. (However, some people do prefer heat during a headache.) The theory is that heat will help increase the blood flow to your head and neck muscles, as well as relaxing them, thus combating muscle contraction headaches.

Cold, on the other hand, is supposed to reduce circulation by constricting the size of the capillaries and arteries. Thus the phase of a migraine marked by the swelling of superficial blood vessels—blood vessels near the surface of your skin, as opposed to those buried deep within your muscles—may be treated with cold.

Cold also reduces the sensitivity of your pain nerve endings, especially those in the back of your head and your upper neck. Since cold travels up the same path to your brain as pain, it overrides the pain impulses. Instead of receiving the message of pain, your brain receives the message of cold.

Finally, cold slows down biological processes. To the extent that your pain is caused by metabolic waste products left in your muscles, it may be eased by slowing down the production of this waste. Since cold decreases the metabolic activity of your muscles, it also decreases muscle spasms that may cause pain.

Regardless of the theories, you should go by your own instincts. Whatever sounds more appealing is probably the right treatment for you.

APPLYING HEAT

Find a position in which your neck is free from strain. The best is to lie on your back, with a low pillow under your knees and a rolled-up towel or small cushion under your neck. The pillow should not be so high that your head is thrown back, but only so that no work is required of your neck muscles. The goal is total relaxation, with all parts of your body supported.

You can also try a sitting position, resting your crossed arms on a table or chair back in front of you, letting your head drop until your forehead is supported by your arms. Be sure your knees are at hip height or above and that your feet are flat on the floor, or on a footstool. Your back should be slumped forward, not slouched back.

There are several methods for applying heat that may work for you. One is simply to sit in the shower in this rest position with hot water beating down on your shoulders and neck. A towel draped in that area may help the heat flow more evenly.

Another method is to use a heating pad on low-intensity, for twenty minutes to an hour. Be sure not to use one for any longer without a long rest period, as otherwise you may damage your skin. A hot water bottle may also bring relief for twenty to sixty minutes. Mentholated lotions will continue the sensation of heat during your "rest" periods.

A soak in a hot tub may also bring deep relaxation, but be sure you are resting your head against a pillow, towel, or cushion, so that your neck may also relax. Again, your head should not be thrown back, but merely supported. If the skin on the back of your neck is wrinkled, your head is arched too far back.

Hot compresses may bring relief. The ideal situation is to have another person apply them, while you relax completely, but you may also apply your own.

Prepare the compresses by folding 100 percent cotton towels into a rectangle of four or five by nineteen inches. Saturate them with hot water and wring them out. Test the temperature—it should be as warm as you can stand it, but not to the point of bringing discomfort.

Once the compresses are prepared, lie down in the position described above, neck and knees supported. Apply one compress behind your neck, another across your forehead, and two over your collarbone, so that your shoulders are covered. After about five minutes, the towels will begin to cool; continue to reheat them and reapply them until you have had about twenty minutes of treatment.

Then give yourself ten minutes of a hot compress placed all over your face, leaving only your nostrils free to breathe. You may wish to combine this physical treatment with one of the relaxation or creative visualization techniques described in Chapter 5, or you may simply wish to savor the heat. In either case, continue to breathe deeply, and allow yourself a moment to savor and stretch when the treatment is done.

APPLYING COLD

You may either wrap some ice cubes in a plastic bag, then in a damp towel; or you may prepare ahead of time by leaving a Styrofoam or paper cup full of water in the freezer, then tearing away the top inch of the cup. Another technique is to leave a damp washcloth in the freezer for about ten minutes and then use it as a cold compress. You can also buy a gel cold pack or cervical ice pillow at the drugstore and leave it in the freezer.

The suboccipital ice pillow (S.I.P.) is a newly marketed product that has been tested at headache centers and found to be as effective in stopping a mild to moderate headache as medication if used early enough in the course of the headache. This device is a soft, comfortable, molded collar/pillow with a thin slit in the back in which you place a frozen gel pack. The collar/pillow then gets fitted around the neck, which ices the back of the skull and the upper neck, affecting critical nerves and muscles to stop the headache.

Apply the cold to the places where you feel pain, to your neck, to the top of your head, or to the upper neck, just below your occipital bone (the bone that sticks out in a little bump on the back of your head). The top of your head is a key acupressure point; that means that many of the nerves that carry messages of pain in this region come together there.

ACUPRESSURE

Acupressure is a variation on the ancient Chinese practice of acupuncture. In acupuncture, a trained practitioner inserts wire-thin needles at key junctures where nerves join muscles. Many people find acupuncture helpful in preventing headache pain and in creating a feeling of well-being generally.

Acupuncture requires a trained practitioner, but acupressure is a technique you may use yourself, either when you feel a headache coming on or when you are in the midst of the pain. You can also teach someone else to administer acupressure to you. Basically, all you need to know is where the pressure points are, and to be willing to press firmly for three minutes. You may not feel anything for the first minute or two, so be patient—wait the full 180 seconds before deciding! If the pressure is causing pain, stop it at once. Never apply pressure to a swollen or infected area.

Here are some key acupressure points that may relieve your headaches: just above the top of the ear, in line with the ear canal; over the bony knobs in the back of the lower part of your skull; just in front of the place where the front of the upper part of your ear attaches to the scalp. There's also a correspondence between your hands and your head, so try pressing the small muscle in the web of your thumb (find it by pressing your thumb toward your palm; it's the muscle that stands out), or the crease where your little finger and your palm join.

MASSAGE

Massage can be used to relieve actual headache pain, or it can be a great way to prevent headaches by relieving tension and improving the circulation. You can get a massage from a professional masseur or masseuse, exchange massages with a friend, or practice self-massage. However, if you have any neck problems, check with your own doctor or headache specialist before trying these techniques.

Naturally, it's most relaxing—and pleasing—to get a massage from someone else. Describing all the techniques of massage is beyond the scope of this book, but there are many excellent books and courses on massage if you wish to explore this field, either alone or with a friend. Many YMCAs and YWCAs offer courses on massage, in addition to holistic or alternative study centers.

To find a professional masseur/masseuse, you might try

advertisements, postings in dance studios, or health food stores, or the advice of a health care practitioner. You may also be able to get a reference from a friend.

Choosing a masseur/masseuse is like choosing a therapist. There are many different schools and philosophies, but in the end, your own instincts are your best guide. Many masseurs and masseuses offer a series of massages as a package; be sure to get one or two trial massages before signing up for more.

If the idea of paying someone to give you a massage and taking one or two hours out of your week to get it sounds unbelievably decadent and extravagant to you, it might be just the experience you need! Perhaps spending some time and money on your own pleasure and relaxation would open up new ways of coping for you, in ways that you least expect.

SELF-MASSAGE

There are many techniques for self-massage, which you can also study further from books, courses, or working with a masseur. Here are a few basic techniques that may be helpful when you feel a headache coming on.

Let your head drop, so that your chin is almost resting on your chest. Put your palms on the back of your head and press, very gently, so that you are stretching out your neck but not straining it. The goal is to relax the muscles in your neck, so begin to imagine them as loose and soft. If they are in reality hard and knotted, don't "fight" them. Think of yourself as working with them, stroking them into softness.

Begin to work on the back of your neck, running your thumbs and fingers down from your skull to your shoulders. From time to time, shake your head gently, from side to side. Think of your head as a balloon, so light that the slightest puff of wind can blow it softly to one side, then the other.

When your neck begins to relax, work your way up over your temples and ears, then back down to your neck. Brace your thumbs against your scalp and rotate them firmly in small circles. You may also find it helpful to press the palms and heels of your hands flat against the sides of your head, with the maximum pressure at the soft points on either side.

Don't press in; pull up, toward the top of your head, and continue to pull for as long as you can.

Alternate these various methods as your instinct dictates, being sure to take little pauses where you again shake your head back and forth or roll it around to keep it loose (see the section on neck rolls, below).

You may also wish to work down to your shoulders. Again, if they feel tight or knotted, don't fight them. Think of yourself as dissolving the tightness, or releasing the softness; find some mental image in which you are working with your body, not against it, and in which your muscles are soft, loose, and warm.

Sometimes this relaxation process seems to release another wave of pain. You may have been braced against some sensation—or some emotion—which your massage is now freeing. If this pain is sudden, sharp, intense, or feels markedly different from any part of a headache you've ever experienced, stop immediately. If, however, it only seems to be a slight intensification of your headache, keep breathing and continue on. Frequently a headache peaks before it passes; you may have to be willing to go through the peak to come out on the other side of the pain.

TREATING YOURSELF FOR EYESTRAIN HEADACHES

People who read for long periods of time, or who work at computer terminals, may find themselves getting headaches due to eyestrain. Technically, it's not the eyes themselves that are being strained; it's the muscles around them, which are used for squinting, blinking, or otherwise reacting to glare or poor light.

Here's an exercise you may find helpful. Remove any lenses you may be wearing and turn down the lights (or go into a dim place, if you are at work). Place your hands over your eyes so that your palms block out the light completely. Then look into the blackness for thirty seconds. Close your eyes again, lower your hands, and then open your eyes slowly.

A little self-massage for an eyestrain headache may be

helpful—but never put any kind of pressure on or near your eyes. Instead, press up on the ridge where your eyebrows are, using your thumbs to push the muscles up. Then work from the top of your nose out to the ends of your eyebrows, moving your thumbs in gentle circles. You may then want to massage your forehead and temples, as well as to try on your temples the press-and-lift technique described above.

SELF-HELP FOR TMJ SYNDROME

As explained in Chapter 2, TMJ syndrome may cause headaches as well as soreness in the jaw. Along with other treatment under the care of your dentist, TMJ specialist, or other health care practitioner, you can try a little self-massage, or get a friend to do this massage for you.

Press your fingers to each tender spot around your ears, holding them there for about ten seconds. Then grab your ears and gently pull them out and down, away from your head. Follow by massaging all around your ear, working your way up to the temples.

You may also wish to work down your neck. Use a downward stroke, but work your way up from the base of your neck to the base of your skull. Then press firmly but gently on the points where your neck and your skull join, and press your thumbs in similar manner against the tender parts on both sides of your jaw. You may wish to pull your jawbone down, lightly, for about twenty seconds. Of course, if any movement causes great or sudden pain, discontinue immediately.

Also, holding a small cylindrical object, such as a pencil, between your teeth may decrease some tension in your jaw muscles. But be careful—hold it, don't bite it!

STRETCHES

Stretching exercises are good for you on several counts. They keep your body flexible, which combats aging. They aid in relaxation and in stimulating circulation, which helps prevent headache. Also, taking stretch breaks from busy or stressful times makes a psychological as well as a physical statement to your system. It can be your way of caring for yourself, of centering and focusing on what's important to you and on your sense of your own power, rather than being swept away in others' demands and needs.

There are a variety of stretches that may be useful to you. Going into all of them is beyond the scope of this book, but the basic stretching routine described here may give you ideas for variations of your own. Or you may take a class in yoga, t'ai chi, dance, or general exercise that offers you additional warmups.

Remember that the point of stretches is to ease the body into long, loose muscles, not to force yourself into an uncomfortable position or to press a muscle into a place it doesn't want to go.

Remember, too, to continue deep breathing throughout the stretching routine. You may need to monitor yourself frequently at first; you'd be surprised at how many people tend to hold their breaths while stretching! In fact, deep, relaxed breathing works with your muscles to stretch your body further. Experiment with how inhaling or exhaling affects your stretches, and make focusing on your breathing a part of your routine.

A BASIC STRETCHING ROUTINE

This routine takes from ten to fifteen minutes, depending on how thorough you are. It's better to move slowly and do a bit less than to rush through it. You can also do parts of this routine during the day to stretch out any body parts that seem tense. You do this stretch in a standing position, wearing flat shoes or barefoot, feet apart, about shoulder width.

Begin with your head. Drop your chin on your chest and let it hang there. Then drop your head back, gently, and let your mouth open. Slowly, continuing to breathe deeply, roll your head around so that your right ear is reaching for your right shoulder. Let your head hang there gently for a moment, then roll front, then left, pausing again. Repeat in the opposite direction. Then roll slowly and continuously to the right for three to five rolls, and repeat an equal number of times in the reverse direction. This is known as a neck roll.

At the end of your neck roll, let your head float up into center upright position. Raise your shoulders, so that they are reaching for your ears. Let them drop and relax completely. Don't throw them down, but let them fall as far as they will go. Inhale (let your breath fall in) on the raise and exhale (let your breath fall out) on the drop. Repeat five or six times.

Then pull your shoulders forward. Feel the difference between raising your shoulders *up* and bringing them *forward.* Pull your shoulders back, so that your shoulder blades are touching. Again, move gently, rather than throwing your body into position. Repeat the forward-back movement five or six times.

Now try bringing one shoulder forward while pushing the other back. Rotate your shoulders around to reverse their position, so that each alternates being front and back. Again, feel the difference between moving just your shoulder and using your whole back or tensing your arms. The goal is to keep all parts of the body completely relaxed except for the part that is moving. Keep in mind the image of how effortlessly the parts of your body are moving.

WORK, POSTURE, AND BODY STRAIN

Many times people at work take a fixed position for hours at a time. The physical stress in doing this contributes greatly to the feeling of psychological tension. Both physical and psychological factors may help to bring on a headache.

The key to preventing this type of headache is to vary your position as frequently as possible. This may be done both while working and by taking breaks. It's also useful to avoid certain positions altogether.

We recently helped a twenty-six-year-old secretary totally rid herself of a chronic headache problem that had her in constant pain. Naturally she was quite depressed because her condition interfered with her social life and plans for the future.

She had a one-year history of moderately severe headache which started in the back of her neck and spread up to include the back half of her head, occasionally reaching up to her temples or spreading to the entire head. The pain was a burning, aching pressure, constant, nonthrobbing with no associated nausea or visual problems. It began three months after she started her present job as a secretary with long hours of sitting in one place, typing, and answering the phone. As the day progressed, so did her neck pain and the resultant headache. On the weekend she was usually pain free.

She began to work with our physical therapist three times per week, concentrating first on posture, then on neck rolls and other exercises specifically designed for her. We suggested a change in her chair, a lumbar support, a change in position every twenty minutes, and a headset telephone. Within six weeks she had no more headaches and now gets a headache only when her boss heaps on the pressure to meet a deadline.

IF YOU WORK AT A DESK

When sitting at a desk, your lower back should always be straight or slumped forward, never slouched back. If you feel yourself settling into a slouch, lift your entire upper body and feel the impulse of energy rising from your lower back up into your head. Ideally, your chair should support your lower back, yet without pressing it forward. If you have no lower back support in the chair you use, rest by leaning forward, so that your weight is over your thighs, not thrust back behind your hips. Take a break every hour or so, even if only for a minute or two.

Your chair should never be so high that your feet can't rest flat on the floor. Your knees should always be at least at hip height, never below. On the other hand, you should be able to reach your desk without strain, with your wrists and elbows more or less level. You may need to use a cushion to raise you if you don't have an adjustable chair.

IF YOU USE A COMPUTER

Video Display Terminals, or VDTs, have been implicated in many health problems, including eyestrain, backache, and headache. You can help combat these health hazards by taking frequent breaks, at least five minutes every one or two hours.

Make the most of these breaks. Do the stretching routine we described above—at least the part where you drop to the floor and then slowly straighten your spine. Breathe deeply. If possible, move to a place where the lighting is different from the area around your terminal. Note wherever you have tension in your body and do gentle stretching or self-massage to combat it. Continue to breathe deeply. You might find it helpful to eat a healthful snack (*not* caffeine or sugar!; see Chapter 7), or, if you have the time, to take a brisk walk in the fresh air, even if it's only two or three laps around the building.

We know that it's frequently difficult to make this kind of time for yourself at work. We understand that many employers are not sympathetic to their workers' need for relaxation. If your workplace is like this, you may have to be creative in taking your breaks, finding ways to do your stretching and breathing in the bathroom or in the corridor of a stairway.

If, on the other hand, the pressure is coming not from your boss, but from yourself, we urge you to consider the benefits of taking time out. You might follow our suggested routine of taking breaks for one week, keeping careful track of exactly how much time you "lose." At the end of the week, note the amount of time. Note also what results you noticed in terms of your productivity, mood, and relations with coworkers, as well as how this change affected your home life. Then compare the time it cost with the amount of time you ordinarily spend with a headache. Use the information to develop the balance between intense work and relaxed breaks that is right for you. We ourselves find that skill at taking breaks allows us greater intensity in our work.

IF YOUR WORK REQUIRES ANOTHER FIXED POSITION

If you have the kind of job that requires standing in one place for a long time, again, we urge you to take brief breaks every hour. Meanwhile, find creative ways to vary your position slightly. Rotate your shoulders, or, if you are hidden behind a counter, do some of the pelvic and torso stretches described above. Don't shift your weight from foot to foot—an evenly balanced posture is best. But do find little ways to keep moving, rather than locking yourself into a fixed position.

Likewise, if you must drive for long hours, breaks are a vital necessity. No one could suggest that you drive in a state of total relaxation; naturally, you must be alert and responsive to traffic and other conditions. But at least adjust the seat so that your legs are comfortably lying loose against the seat, rather than stretched out. Be sure you don't have to stretch to reach the steering wheel, and use a pillow or lumbar roll to support your back if the car seat does not provide enough support. As with people who work at desks, keep your weight up and your spine straight. For a change, slump forward rather than slouching back. Don't drive more than one or two hours at a time without taking a brief break that consists of walking and stretching outside of the car.

EXERCISE AND YOUR DAILY ROUTINE

Probably the single most important thing you can do of all the suggestions made in this chapter is to take up some regular aerobic exercise: walking, running, bicycling, swimming, or an aerobic sport, such as tennis or racquetball. Although some people have health reasons for not engaging in some of these activities, almost anyone can walk at a brisk pace for fifteen to twenty minutes a day, four days a week. Just this addition of exercise into your routine could make an enormous difference in how you feel. (If you have any doubts about your ability to do any form of exercise, including walking, check with your physician before beginning. If you notice any ill effects, stop immediately and again, check with your doctor.)

Exercise has both physical and emotional benefits. It improves circulation because your body—especially your heart—develops extra capillaries in order to respond to the new activity. Thus your tissues are served with more oxygen, and waste products are more efficiently removed from your muscles. And your circulation is improved by the so-called "collateral circulation" provided by the extra capillaries.

Exercise also saves your heart a great deal of work. Every time your thigh muscles contract and relax, as they do in exercise, they pump blood back into the heart, taking some of the strain off the heart muscle itself. Exercise also keeps blood moving throughout your body, rather than "pooling" in one place.

Your lungs and your chest also benefit from regular exercise. The circulation of blood through your lungs is improved, and your breathing leads your diaphragm to "massage" your inner organs of the upper abdomen, such as the stomach, liver, pancreas, and spleen. Deep breathing also opens your rib cage, which improves your posture, easing the strain on your back.

The chemical benefits of exercise also affect your emotions. We believe that intense exercise helps produce endorphins. These morphine-like chemicals produced by your brain create a sense of well-being and also raise your pain threshold. There is also some sort of effect on your sense of well-being that comes from what is called your kinesthetic sense, which is your muscles' awareness of movement. Moderately vigorous rhythmic exercise may produce a "runner's high" and make you feel good for hours.

Moderate, regular exercise is better than a killer workout once a week, since your goal is to raise the entire level of your body's functioning. People who jog or walk briskly on a regular basis have reported dramatic improvements in their headaches, as well as curative effects on sleep problems, depression, and anxiety. Even if it's just the placebo effect, it seems to work!

If you prefer an exercise regime of lifting weights, we caution you to work carefully with a trainer, so that you aren't inadvertently taking positions that are stressing and contracting muscles that may be involved in your headaches. Weight lifting tends to contract the muscles, whereas aerobic exercise loosens and lengthens them. In fact, vigorous weight lifting can even cause headaches. We also remind you that weight lifting, however demanding, is not aerobic exercise, and so should be supplemented by walking, running, swimming, or some similar activity.

Recent scientific research shows that moderate aerobic exercise for twenty to thirty minutes three times a week prolongs life and decreases the likelihood of certain kinds of cancer and heart problems. Interestingly, this particular benefit to life span and the heart doesn't seem to increase as you do more exercise. However, an exercise schedule that involves some aerobic activity—walking, running, swimming, and so on—four or five times a week does seem to make an appreciable difference in reducing headaches and promoting a general sense of well-being.

[7]

NOURISHING YOURSELF:
DIET AND HEADACHE

MEETING YOUR UNIQUE
NUTRITIONAL NEEDS

EVERY HUMAN BODY is different. Your body has its own
unique chemistry. Your pancreas releases insulin to metabolize blood sugar at its own specific rate. Your adrenal
glands release adrenaline in response to their own set of
physical and emotional signals. Your biochemistry interacts
with various foods, with alcohol and caffeine, with vitamins
and minerals, in its own special way.

Of course, every human body also operates according
to certain principles. The purpose of this chapter is to give
you the basic information you need to become aware of
how your body works and how this affects your headaches.
We'll cover various dietary triggers that set off headaches
in some people, as well as explain an interesting theory
that relates migraine and other headaches to low blood
sugar and offers a corresponding way of eating that has
been startlingly effective in reducing headache. We'll suggest a method whereby you can experiment with different
foods, vitamins, and eating habits, to see which methods
work best for you. And we'll give you our own suggestions
for good eating habits that counteract headache.

After that, it's up to you! Working either alone or with
a nutritionist, you can develop the body awareness that will
help you determine what you need to eat and what you

need to avoid to reduce and prevent your headaches. In our experience, diet can be a powerful tool for good health—and an inappropriate diet is often at the root of many headaches. If you're willing to become aware of your eating habits and to change them, you may be able to eliminate most or all of your headaches.

DIET AND HEADACHE

When we say "diet" in this book, we are referring to everything that you put into your system. In addition to food and beverages, diet includes alcohol, recreational drugs, prescription drugs, off-the-shelf medications, cigarettes, other forms of tobacco, and caffeine. All of these substances affect your body's biochemistry. All of them demand certain responses from your organs and your glands. Some of these responses may trigger the processes that give you headaches.

Sometimes a substance will give you a headache in one circumstance and not in another. Many women, for example, are especially susceptible to headaches during the week before or the week of their periods. (For more information on menstrual migraine, see Chapter 8.) For these women, a chocolate bar may be safe the rest of the month and a headache trigger during the premenstrual week.

If you've been keeping up a healthy regimen of aerobic exercise, you may find that you can take a glass of wine or two with impunity. If you've missed your running for a few days, however, and you can feel that your muscles are knotted up in stress, the same amount of wine may set off a terrible migraine.

Throughout this book, we've talked about headaches and their triggers as an interactive process, in which many related factors influence one another to arrive at the final outcome. Nowhere is this more true than with your diet. Simply cutting down on caffeine, for example, may drastically change your susceptibility to other foods that, while you are drinking three cups of coffee a day, are sure to set off a migraine. Possibly you have a long-term vitamin deficiency, probably of one of the B vitamins, which, when corrected, may affect your vulnerability to other headache triggers. Perhaps eating a sugary brownie sets off your headache reaction. But eating that brownie with some protein—say, a glass of milk—may cause you to react quite differently.

It's also possible that there are some foods, beverages, or substances that will inevitably set off a headache, regardless of what else you do. And your reactions to foods and other substances may change over time. Foods that were once "safe" become headache triggers; foods that used to be poison may now be eaten occasionally in small quantities.

Why are we telling you this? Because in this chapter, we are going to give you information that may challenge your idea of what a healthy diet is and what's acceptable for you to eat. And this may mean giving up some of your favorite foods, at least temporarily, in exchange for cutting down your headaches.

Most of us have strong emotional attachments to food. We associate favorite foods with special occasions, loved ones, comforting ourselves, childhood memories. We want to be able to eat in restaurants and fast-food joints with our colleagues, to serve our children the same food we grew up eating ourselves, to indulge ourselves with a few drinks at a party or with a fragrant cup of coffee in the morning. Learning that these reliable pleasures may be giving us some of the worst pain of our lives isn't easy.

Changing to a diet that may be different from those of many of our friends and family isn't easy, either. So we want to encourage you to keep an open mind. The information in this chapter is to help you see and feel for yourself the relationship between what you put into your mouth and what happens "inside" your head. In the end, only you can know which diet is best for you.

HOW YOUR DIGESTIVE SYSTEM WORKS

When you put a substance into your mouth, the enzymes in your saliva begin right away to break it down.

When you swallow, the food passes through a long tube called the esophagus, into your stomach. Your stomach responds to the substance by releasing more digestive chemicals, which further break down the food.

From your stomach, the food passes into your small intestine, where it undergoes more chemical changes. As a result of the enzymes and chemicals released by your body, a food substance has by now been broken down into its component parts: carbohydrates (a combination of carbon and water found in every living thing), fat, protein, vitamins, minerals, and waste.

All of the components except waste pass through the wall of your small intestine into your bloodstream. The blood then carries the nutrients to the different parts of your body, where they are used to fuel your energy, and to repair and renew your tissue, bones, nerves, and muscles.

The components that can't be used right away are stored. Some of them are stored as body fat. That's why, if you are taking in more food than your body can use, you gain weight. Another portion of this food is stored as glycogen, a substance that can be converted into glucose, or blood sugar. In order for you to feel fit and healthy, the glucose in your blood has to be at a certain level. If it falls below that level, your body will convert glycogen into glucose.

The parts of the food you can't use are known as waste. They pass into your large intestine, and from there into your rectum, which expels them regularly. If you are eating the wrong foods, or if there is some other body problem, the waste may rot or decompose within your large intestine. In addition to any toxins (poisons, or unhealthy substances for your body) that may have been in the waste to begin with, toxins are created by this putrefaction process.

Sometimes these toxins are also reabsorbed into the blood. Then, when the blood passes through the liver, the liver tries to cleanse it, and it too may become toxic. That's why drinking alcohol puts such a strain on your liver. In trying to clean the alcohol (which it experiences as toxic) out of the bloodstream, the liver may develop cellular damage. Medication, recreational drugs, nicotine, pesticides that may be clinging to fresh fruits and vegetables, hormones that may have been added to cattle and poultry, rancid oil in snack food, or other spoiled food are all toxins that can have a bad effect on parts of your body.

Your liver is interrelated with parts of your endocrine (hormonal) system. This is the system that determines how much of your body's stored food energy should be converted into a usable form of energy. As you can see, if your liver is under a strain, it won't be able to perform either function properly: neither cleansing the blood of toxins, nor regulating the conversion of stored energy to blood sugar. Toxins in your blood and inappropriate levels of blood sugar may both contribute to headaches.

One aspect of a healthy diet, then, is giving up or cutting back on foods that put an unnatural strain on your liver. Probably most people in the United States eat in such a way as to strain their livers, but those of us with headaches have additional evidence that we may be doing so. Even if we are eating the same diet as someone who does not get headaches, this diet may be putting a strain on our particular systems.

CHOICES FOR A HEALTHIER DIET

Many doctors believe that the following choices will generally make for a healthier diet with more respect for your liver. Since very little scientific research has been done in this area, we hesitate to make any definite pronouncements. But we thought you should know about some of these theories of diet. No one would suggest that you convert your eating habits overnight. But you may want to experiment with these choices, possibly making one substitution a week, just to see how it makes you feel:

- no medication for one month (This applies to off-the-shelf analgesics or unnecessary medications. Any standard medication given by a physician should be taken under medical supervision.)
- relaxation methods instead of alcohol or drugs
- juices, seltzer, or spring water instead of soda (even artificially sweetened, decaffeinated soda)
- herb teas instead of caffeinated drinks (even decaf-

feinated coffee); decrease caffeine gradually over two weeks
- organic or homegrown vegetables instead of those sprayed with pesticides.
- homemade snacks, nuts, seeds, or hot-air popcorn instead of prepared foods

CANDIDA ALBICANS: A DIGESTIVE PROBLEM

One common though little known microorganism that is affected by nutrition is known as *Candida albicans*. This yeastlike fungus is normally found in all human bodies, where it is kept in check by certain bacteria that are usually also present. However, sometimes taking antibiotics can destroy "good" bacteria as well as "bad" ones. In some people, if the bacteria that control the yeast are destroyed by antibiotics, there may be an overgrowth of *Candida albicans* as the result. Other factors that may dispose you to *Candida* overgrowth are diabetes, general debility, and nutritional deficiencies.

The symptoms of this candidiasis are exhaustion, drowsiness, difficulties with bowel movement (both constipation and diarrhea), stomach pain, and headaches. Sweets, wheat, yeast products (such as doughnuts, coffee cakes, and breads), and alcohol (especially beer and other "yeasty" drinks) can aggravate the condition.

If you think you have *Candida albicans*, you should work with a doctor or nutritionist to develop your own diet to combat it. Generally, people with this syndrome follow a nutritional program that focuses on poultry, fish, rice, millet, oats, and other vegetables, possibly with supplements of vitamins, minerals, hydrochloric acid, acidophilus, and antifungal nutrients.

FOOD ALLERGIES

There's a lot of controversy about this area. Some experts believe that food allergies play a very small role in headache, and in a person's health generally. Others believe that many of us have minor, unnoticed allergies to food—which translate themselves into headaches and other "minor" difficulties. Since many allergens (substances that set off someone's allergies) are normally considered healthy—for example, wheat, corn, and dairy products—we don't realize that they may be causing problems for us.

As we've said before, each person's body is unique. The food that may be healthy for one may be an allergen for another. Common allergens include: shellfish, dairy products, eggs, corn, peanuts, wheat, rye, barley, citrus fruits, onions, vegetables in the nightshade family (tomatoes, potatoes, eggplant, and bell peppers), preservatives, additives and artificial coloring, tobacco, alcohol, drugs, chocolate, and sugar.

If you wish to explore the possibility that you have some mild or subtle food allergy, you may wish to work with a nutritionist to identify possible problem areas. In our opinion, the great majority of headaches are not caused by food allergies. However, chemicals in foods can cause blood vessels to react in such a way as to cause a headache. If all other treatments have failed and allergies are being considered, a consultation with an allergist may be appropriate.

DAIRY PRODUCTS

Dairy products are milk and the products made from it, including cheese, yogurt, cream cheese, sour cream, and ice cream. Although sinusitis isn't usually a cause of headache, dairy products may put a strain on your sinuses. They cause you to produce increased amounts of phlegm and mucus, which blocks your sinuses. This may cause you additional discomfort during your headache attacks; or you may have an allergy to dairy products that sets off a headache.

Dairy products do include the important mineral calcium. However, you can get adequate calcium from green leafy vegetables, nuts, grains, and supplements. If you frequently feel that your head is clogged, or that sinus problems accompany your headaches, you might try eliminating dairy products from your diet completely for two to four weeks and noting the result. You might decide to eliminate them permanently, you might avoid them at stressful times or around the time of your period, or you might simply cut down on dairy products.

HEADACHE AND HYPOGLYCEMIA

Another trigger of headache pain is *hypoglycemia,* or low blood sugar. In *diabetes* (or *hyperglycemia*) blood sugar levels rise too high, since the pancreas is unable to produce enough *insulin,* the substance that breaks down blood sugar and stores it in a usable form. Hypoglycemics have the opposite problem: their pancreas is overacuve. It produces too much insulin, which drives their blood sugar down below an acceptable level.

There is a good deal of controversy about how to use the term "hypoglycemia." Many doctors recognize only a strict definition of this syndrome, diagnosed only by certain criteria on a five-hour glucose tolerance test.

However, there may be degrees of hypoglycemia. If you feel anxious, irritable, depressed, confused, or extremely moody after missing a meal; if missing a meal causes you to have poor memory, dizziness, fatigue, tremors, or cold sweats; if you find yourself continually craving sugar and other sweet things; or if skipping a meal or eating later than usual seems to bring on a headache, you may have relative hypoglycemia (a much milder form of the condition).

If you're beginning to suspect you're hypoglycemic, you can ask your doctor or nutritionist for a glucose tolerance test. This is the same test that is given to diabetics, to see how their bodies respond to changes in blood sugar.

What should happen in a healthy body is that blood sugar goes up after a person eats, stimulating the production of insulin, which then drives the blood sugar level

192 / HEADACHE RELIEF

back down to normal. In a diabetic, the blood sugar level does not return to normal within two hours, because not enough insulin is being produced. In a hypoglycemic, on the other hand, the blood sugar tends to fall considerably below normal, as too much insulin is produced.

If you're taking a glucose tolerance test, be careful. The normal test is taken over a period of two hours, long enough to reveal the presence of diabetes. But two hours is not long enough to reveal the presence of hypoglycemia. After two hours, a hypoglycemic's body has just about gotten his or her blood sugar level down to normal. But, because of the excess of insulin produced, the next three hours will see blood sugar going down *below* normal. Those three hours are a crucial testing time for hypoglycemia. Therefore, your doctor should order a five-hour glucose tolerance test.

Since patients with this syndrome may still show up normal on a glucose tolerance test, the lab test is not very important, except for documentation purposes. If the syndrome we're describing seems familiar to you, try the modifications we suggest, which in any case can do you no harm. If they seem to work for you, then you've found an effective way to deal with your mood disturbances and your headaches, regardless of the diagnosis.

How Hypoglycemia Leads to Headaches

When you eat a starch (e.g., pasta, bread, potatoes, rice, or other grains) or a sugar (e.g., processed sugar, honey, corn syrup, or a fruit containing its own sugars), these components are broken down via a number of steps, and are eventually absorbed into your bloodstream as glucose, or blood sugar. Your network of blood vessels then carries blood, with its oxygen and glucose throughout your body.

All parts of your body, including your brain, need glucose and oxygen in order to function. Therefore, the level of glucose in your blood is extremely important to your body. A variety of organs and glands are involved in monitoring this level, since it's so crucial to your functioning. The pituitary, thyroid, adrenal glands, pancreas, and liver all make sure you have the level of glucose that you need.

When you eat—or when you ingest processed sugar,

alcohol, tobacco, caffeine, marijuana, or cocaine—your blood sugar level goes up. This alerts your pancreas to produce more insulin, to combat the high level of glucose.

How does insulin do this? It helps glucose cross from the blood through the walls of your blood vessels into your tissues.

What if there's too much glucose to be absorbed into your tissues? Then the insulin "tells" your liver to convert some of the glucose in your blood into *glycogen,* the body's form of stored glucose. This glycogen will be available to your body when your blood sugar level drops again. If you exercise, for example, you're burning up energy, or blood sugar. So your body converts some of its stored energy, or glycogen, to make up the difference.

Eventually, of course, you'll have to eat something to replenish the lost energy. But a healthy body can get along for quite some time on its stored energy.

For the hypoglycemic and the diabetic, however, this process goes awry. A normal pancreas will get blood sugar down to 70 to 110 milligrams (mg) percent (that is, per 100 milliliters of blood). A diabetic's pancreas can only get blood sugar down to 130–300 mg percent, which means that the food he or she eats isn't getting turned into energy by the body. That's why diabetics have to take extra injections of insulin when their blood sugar is too high.

A hypoglycemic, on the other hand, has an overactive pancreas. It produces so much insulin that the body's blood sugar drops down to 40–50 mg percent. Too much glucose is leaving the blood vessels for the body's tissues. There may be a greater degree of hypoglycemia after eating, and especially after drinking alcohol, eating foods that contain sugar, or getting high. Suddenly, the body's blood sugar level is too low.

Your body experiences this as an emergency. The new chain of events that's set in motion is thus biologically similar to what happens when you're under stress—that is, when you perceive a danger that must be met by "fight or flight." Your body is signaling your brain that it may not function properly without more blood sugar—and soon!

In trying to get its glucose level back up, the body

stimulates the adrenal glands (after all, you're facing an "emergency"). Among other substances, your adrenals produce *catecholamines*. These chemical neurotransmitters constrict the blood vessels to get blood traveling through your body with more force, "visiting" the sugar-starved areas more quickly in order to bring what little blood sugar is left to your body's tissues.

The catecholamines also raise your body temperature, blood pressure, and pulse rate; cause shallow breathing; and generally produce the "fight or flight" feeling of mobilizing for a frightening emergency. Hence the symptoms we described above—headaches; a feeling of panic, irritability, or despair; and difficulties with memory, concentration, and balance.

The blood vessel constriction can't continue forever, of course. So it triggers an opposite reaction, the production of prostaglandins. Some of these chemicals dilate your blood vessels—which in turn may produce the throbbing pain of migraine.

Interestingly, when migraineurs were given a shot of insulin, they reacted by developing a migraine. People without migraines were given a double dose of insulin, and got no headaches. And only about half of all hypoglycemics get migraine. So, even though we have some idea of *how* blood sugar is related to headache pain, we still don't know *why* the process we've described leads to headaches in some cases and not in others. Once again, some people seem to have a biological predisposition to have headaches —but some combination of other factors must trigger this tendency. You yourself may have noticed that sometimes your hypoglycemic reaction includes a headache, whereas other times you can miss a meal with little more than a slight feeling of annoyance. Women migraineurs report that they're especially likely to get headaches from missed meals around the time of their periods.

EASING THE HYPOGLYCEMIC REACTION

Major swings in blood sugar are primarily caused by ingesting processed sugar, as well as alcohol, drugs, and caffeine (for a further explanation of how alcohol and caffeine affect your blood sugar, see the sections on these substances below). That's because processed sugars (including honey, maple syrup, dextrose, and corn syrup) have no other nutrients to ease the conversion of the food into glucose. Processed sugar is converted into glucose almost immediately—hence the rapid overreaction of your insulin-producing pancreas.

The best way to control a hypoglycemic reaction is to avoid processed sugar completely, as well as all foods that contain it. Cookies, cakes, ice cream, and candy all contain huge amounts of processed sugar. Many canned, frozen, and otherwise preserved foods also contain sugar, corn syrup, or dextrose, even such "nonsweet" foods as canned soup or frozen vegetables.

If you're not willing to give up sugar completely, we suggest cutting down on the foods you eat that contain processed sugar, as well as never eating sweet foods on an empty stomach. Starch and sugar are converted into glucose, while protein is converted into amino acids. So eating some protein first or at the same time gives your body two tasks instead of one, thus slowing the rate at which the sweet food is converted to glucose. The more slowly this conversion takes place, the more you will avoid a "rush" and so avoid triggering a hypoglycemic reaction.

Eating Tips for Hypoglycemics

Naturally, we recommend that you avoid all foods containing processed sugar, including honey, dextrose, and corn syrup. (While honey may seem like a "natural" ingredient, most bees are fed corn syrup or some other sugary produce, which makes honey as bad as sugar from a hypoglycemic's point of view.) Cutting back on the following items will help reduce your tendency to hypoglycemic reactions: sugar, honey, soft drinks, juices to which sugar has been added, canned or frozen fruit, vegetables to which sugar has been added, baked beans, baked goods, potato chips, pretzels, ice cream, dates, raisins, dried fruit, caffeinated beverages, alcohol, and recreational drugs.

As with our other diet suggestions, we recommend cutting these items completely out of your diet for at least a month, noting the reaction, then gradually adding items back, one at a time, also noting your reactions. That way, you can see for yourself how these substances affect your body, and decide for yourself whether the pleasant taste or social experience is worth the aftereffects. You may also notice that these foods affect your body differently under different circumstances, depending on the rest of your diet, your general level of fitness and stress, and, for women, the time of the month.

On the other hand, we recommend eating plenty of the following foods: lean meats, fish, and poultry; green leafy vegetables; cucumbers; squash; soybeans and related products (like tofu); nuts, seeds, and peanut butter; fresh fruits (with citrus in moderation); potatoes; and whole grains, including whole grain bread. Even white flour products, such as pasta, have enough other nutrients so that they will not produce the hypoglycemic reaction that sugar or a sugary product will. A whole wheat honey-sweetened coffee cake is far worse for you than a plate of spaghetti.

You should also try to eat as regularly as possible, making especially sure to have some protein and a carbohydrate, preferably a whole grain containing the outermost bran layers and the inner germ, bread, pasta, or cold or hot unsweetened cereal first thing in the morning. Even if you aren't eating sugar, your pancreas is working overtime to produce insulin if you're a hypoglycemic. Thus your blood sugar level is automatically being brought down more quickly than other people's—and you need to restore it with some protein and a carbohydrate.

Some hypoglycemics need to eat a light snack—say, crackers and mild cheese (cottage or American)—just before going to bed, so that their blood sugar doesn't drop too fast during the night. Some extreme cases even need to set their alarms, wake up, and eat a few crackers during the night.

If you rebalance your diet, cutting out processed sugars and eating frequent, small, high protein meals with some carbohydrates, you may notice a general improvement and an increase in your ability to tolerate delayed meals. In any case, increasing your body awareness will help you learn how to eat something *before* the danger period begins.

Many hypoglycemics carry with them protein-carbohydrate snacks, such as cheese and crackers, so that they never feel "at the mercy" of a sudden drop in blood sugar.

MEDICATION AND INSULIN

Some prescribed medications actually stimulate the production of insulin, which increases your chance of headaches if you are hypoglycemic. Ask your doctor about the possible effects of the following medications: bishydroxy-coumarin, calcium gluconate, chlorpromazine, corticosteroids, ibuprofen (found in Advil), nitrobenzodiazepine derivative, oxyquinazoline, oxytetracycline, phenylbutazone, propoxyphene (found in Darvon), salicylates (found in aspirin), sulfisoxazole. An equivalent substitute is usually available.

WHAT ABOUT ARTIFICIAL SWEETENERS?

Saccharin contains nothing that will stimulate your insulin production—but many studies suggest that it increases your risk of cancer. The latest artificial sweeteners, Nutrasweet and Equal, are both forms of aspartame, made of aspartic acid and the methyl ester of phenylalanine. These substances are actually amino acids and have little or no relation to your glucose level. In small amounts, they should not trigger insulin production. However, they too may pose other health risks.

Generally, artificial sweeteners stimulate your appetite for the real thing. Some studies have shown that artificial sweeteners actually stimulate people to gain weight, as they are used with various metabolism-lowering diets. In general, we don't recommend the use of artificial sweeteners—but it's true that they won't trigger an insulin reaction! However, some people do seem to get headaches from aspartame, even though the manufacturer denies that it happens. We suggest taking it out of your diet.

HEADACHE TRIGGERS AND CRAVINGS

The following foods seem to be headache triggers for many people: pork; game and organ meats (including liver, kidney, sweetbreads, and brains); smoked and cured, aged, and packaged meat (including corned beef, cold cuts, salami, hot dogs, ham, and sausage); herring, caviar, and smoked fish; vinegar; pickled and fermented foods; aged cheese (such as cheddar, Brie, and Gruyère); products high in yeasts and tyramines (including doughnuts, coffee cakes, and breads, especially hot, fresh bread); chocolate; sugar and all products made with processed sugar or corn syrup; citrus fruits in large quantities; figs; cream; sour cream; yogurt; the pods of lima beans, navy beans, and peas; flavor enhancers such as MSG; caffeine; and alcoholic beverages, especially red wine.

Again, we suggest either working with a nutritionist or an elimination diet; Cut all of the above foods out of your diet for one month. Then add one food at a time, noting its effect on you and your headaches. (If eliminating these foods for a month has no effect on your headaches, then you should certainly be working with a doctor.)

FOOD CRAVINGS, FOOD ALLERGIES, AND HEADACHES

You may even discover, after giving up some of the above substances for a month, that they no longer appeal to you—even if formerly, you used to get terrific cravings for them. Food cravings seem to be a part of some people's headache cycles, especially those with menstrual migraines. (For more about menstrual migraines, see Chapter 8.)

There are a variety of theories about food cravings. One suggests that many of us develop addictions to certain foods. Both coffee and sugar produce certain effects on our body, such as waking us up or giving us a rush of energy. When these substances are withdrawn, our body can't produce the same effect by itself, which leads to a powerful craving as the body tries to get the old effect back. Even though these foods may be making us sick, the body has learned to want them.

Another theory of food cravings is that the brain changes that produce our headaches also affect the hypothalamus, or appetite center. Thus the cravings are not a cause of our headache, but an effect of the same process that produces it. This theory is supported by the fact that many women get cravings around the time of their periods, which is also a time when they are especially prone to migraine.

Possibly, both factors are involved. Changes in our brain may set up a craving for food that will speed up or intensify the headache process. Or a brain change is a precondition for a headache—and a craving—but eating the food is the final factor that pushes the change "over the edge." Thus, if you are feeling on the verge of a headache, the caffeine, sugar, or alcohol that you crave might make that headache a reality, whereas a quick snack of protein and carbohydrates (say, some mild cheese—cottage or American—and crackers, or a handful of peanuts) might reverse the process.

We certainly don't mean to imply that every food craving is an unhealthy one. Some cravings are your body's way of telling you what you need. Armed with the information in this chapter, and with your own experience, you can learn to feel the difference between a craving you should listen to and one that will trigger a headache.

THE DIFFERENT TYPES OF HEADACHE TRIGGERS

We've given you a long list of headache triggers. Here are some more details about the different categories they fall into, and more examples of the foods in each category.

AMINES
Amines are biological substances that help your brain and blood vessels to function. Some of them are produced by your body; others must be supplied by eating other substances.

As we saw in Chapter 1, the brain functions by electrical currents that travel throughout the brain, the spinal cord, and the peripheral nerves, which carry messages from the brain. The electricity is generated through chemical reactions between your cells and various chemical substances that you take into your body, through eating, drinking, or smoking. Thus, eating a hamburger, smoking a cigarette, or drinking a shot of whiskey all conduct different chemicals into your body, setting off various chemical reactions that in turn affect your brain.

The chemical substances that affect your nerve cells are known as *neurotransmitters*. We don't completely understand how these neurotransmitters act within the brain, but we do know that there are various types of neurotransmitters, each with its own function. The neurotransmitters that seem most important for headache problems are called biogenic amines, that is, amines that your body itself has generated.

These biogenic amines seem to help regulate sleeping, moods, blood pressure, and heart rate. Variations in amine levels seem to be related to psychiatric and neurological disorders, including schizophrenia, depression, Parkinson's disease, and Huntington's disease. Amines also seem to be implicated in migraine headaches.*

Many foods contain amines, which, as we've said, are necessary for the brain's continued functioning. However, too high a level of amines may have an adverse effect on migraineurs and on others with headaches. Tyramine causes blood vessels to start the constriction process that leads to migraine and also releases prostaglandins, which further affect the vessels.

A headache trigger may work in a variety of ways. Some triggers set off a headache under any circumstances, particularly alcohol. Others must be eaten in large quantities. Sometimes stressful times or menstrual timing will add to a trigger's likelihood to produce a headache, whereas regular exercise or a calmer time make a trigger less potent.

Some of these triggers are more potent than others.

---

* Some studies suggest that people with migraines are also prone to depression. In addition to the possibility that the repeated experience of apparently uncontrollable pain might foster the sense of helplessness and despair associated with depression, it's also possible that amines are a biological link between depression and migraine.

Sugar, chocolate, fatty foods, and citrus fruits (especially oranges) are among the most often cited headache triggers.

The one substance that almost everyone agrees is dangerous for headache people is alcohol. Red wine, brandy, and sherry are almost guaranteed to give you a headache. Other forms of alcohol are also likely triggers. We'll deal with alcohol in more detail below, as well; for now, let's just note that alcohol shows up as a headache trigger on several counts—for its amine content; its effect on your liver; its content of sugar, malt, and yeast; and its role as a dilator of your blood vessels.

NITRITES

Nitrites have been used for centuries to preserve meat, going back to the early Romans and Asians. In our preservative-happy age, it's used even more frequently, in such foods as the following: canned ham, corned beef, smoked fish, salami, bologna, sausage, pepperoni, summer sausage, bacon, and the ever-popular hot dog.

Every year, some 12 billion pounds of nitrite are added to our food supply. The compound acts to prevent botulism, a potentially fatal disease that comes from improperly preserved food. It also gives meat a special "cured" taste, and turns it red or pink.

Nitrite seems to trigger blood vessel dilation in the human body. Sometimes, we take medical advantage of this effect, as when we prescribe nitroglycerin for treatment in heart disease. However, this dilation may also cause a headache in some people.

The nitrite headache is usually felt in both temples, as a dull, throbbing pain (the result of swelling blood vessels). If you are going to get a nitrite headache, it will probably come on within thirty minutes of the time you eat the nitrite-containing food.

Nitrites may also combine with some amines to form nitrosamines. There's some evidence that this substance causes cancer, although so far, the research on this topic has only been done on animals. Humans may react differently.

MSG

Another food additive that may cause headaches is monosodium glutamate (MSG), used to enhance the flavor of food, and used most frequently in Chinese cooking. The food enhancer Accent also contains large quantities of MSG.

MSG is actually a natural component of protein. It's chemically related to an important neurotransmitter in the brain, GABA (gamma-aminobutyric acid), which would explain why eating large quantities of it would affect brain and nervous system activity.

GABA, in turn, may release acetylcholine, which stimulates muscle function. Acetylcholine may also keep the brain cells from absorbing enough blood sugar, which sets off a hypoglycemic reaction (for more information, see the section on hypoglycemia above).

Some people experience a variety of symptoms when they eat large amounts of MSG, particularly on an empty stomach: sweating, anxiety, tightness and burning in the chest and stomach, flushing, mood changes, tingling in the hands, pain in the neck and eyes—and, of course, headache. An MSG headache features pounding pain over the temples and a sense of tightness, like a squeezing headband, around the forehead.

The reaction usually occurs within fifteen to twenty-five minutes after eating the MSG. However, if you've eaten non-MSG-containing food before eating the MSG, the MSG's absorption into your bloodstream is slowed. The symptoms may be delayed, or may not occur at all.

Some 10 to 25 percent of the population may be sensitive to MSG and its effects. Possibly, headaches may be the only sign of this sensitivity, without the other symptoms. Yet some 20,000 tons of MSG are added to our food each year. Here are some of the items that include this product: many TV dinners; self-basting turkeys; instant gravy; processed meats; canned and instant soup; dry-roasted nuts; some potato chips; tenderizers and seasonings, such as Accent, Lawry's Seasoned Salt, and so on.

These days, most Chinese restaurants will leave out the MSG if you ask them to. Eliminating the substance from the rest of your diet will require a careful reading of labels.

ICE CREAM HEADACHES

Some people experience a sudden headache as they take a bite of ice cream. Possibly the pain will come in from the throat or face, rather than their head. A dull, throbbing pain seems to radiate throughout the head, originating deep behind the bridge of the nose. The pain lasts for only a few minutes.

We don't completely understand what causes this event, though we imagine it has to do with the sudden cold shock to the warm tissues of the mouth and throat. The discomfort is referred from the mouth to branches of various cranial nerves: the fifth, which carries sensations from the front of the mouth, and the ninth, which carries sensations from the back of the throat. (See Chapter 1 for a more complete explanation of referred pain.) Cold may also affect the carotid arteries in the back of the throat.

There's no permanent treatment for an ice cream headache, but they're fairly easy to avoid: Allow the ice cream to become a little less cold, and/or allow small bits to melt inside your mouth, to cool off those warm tissues and make the temperature change somewhat less extreme when it goes down.

SALT

Although we don't have a clear explanation of just how salt causes headaches, many people believe that it can be a provocative factor. It seems to aggravate high blood pressure, which is correlated with headache, especially migraine. Salt may be found in soy sauce and tamari sauce, as well as in most packaged and prepared foods. Many nutritionists believe that sea salt is more healthful than the other type, but caution that in any case, our diets contain far too much of this substance, which may even be found in packaged sweet things.

CHOCOLATE

This addictive treat has four headache-provoking components, which together make for a powerful headache trigger. The ground cacao seeds that give chocolate its dark flavor have a slight hypoglycemic effect. This effect is multiplied when combined with the sweeteners in chocolate, which have their own hypoglycemic effect. Chocolate also contains some caffeine, which, as we shall see, is a third headache trigger. Lastly, chocolate contains phenylethyl-amine, a substance that affects blood vessels and so may trigger a headache.

SMOKING

As you're no doubt already aware, smoking has a very destructive effect on your heart, lungs, and blood vessels. The nicotine in tobacco is a vasoconstrictor, like ergotam-ine. Thus, like ergotamine, your body comes to depend upon it to keep your blood vessels constricted. As you become ever dependent upon nicotine, your body needs ever higher amounts to keep the blood vessels constricted, producing a rebound effect whereby smoking may contribute to your headaches. It also causes instability of blood vessels.

In addition, smokers have high levels of carbon monoxide and carboxyhemoglobin in their blood, substances that displace oxygen and cause a consequent lack of oxygen in the brain. Lack of oxygen causes your blood vessels to dilate in an attempt to carry more blood to the brain—which again may trigger a headache.

On the other hand, since your body has become dependent upon nicotine for vasoconstriction, if you stop smoking, you may also go through a period of withdrawal during which you get headaches. Sooner or later, of course, your body becomes accustomed to doing without nicotine.

In addition, smoking increases your risk of cancer and heart disease, as well as other circulatory problems, such as stroke. Migraineurs who smoke have increased this risk—and migraineurs who smoke and take birth control pills or other hormone treatments are facing a triple threat. That's because all three conditions—getting migraine, taking hormones, and smoking—have a potentially detrimental effect on blood vessel activity.

How does this work? We know that some migraineurs have spasms in the blood vessels that carry blood to their brains. Smoking constricts these and other blood vessels, while the estrogen in birth control pills or other hormone treatments causes spasms in the arteries. Hence the triple threat—spasms in constricted arteries carrying blood to the brain. To make matters worse, some of these patients could be treated with ergotamine, a medication that constricts blood vessels even further.

HEADACHES AND CAFFEINE

Although caffeine is actually a powerful drug, we don't tend to think of it in those terms. Caffeine can be found in coffee, tea, chocolate, soft drinks, and in some painkillers, including Anacin, Excedrin, and most "sinus headache"

TABLE 7.1

CAFFEINE IN FOOD AND MEDICINE

SOURCE	ESTIMATED CAFFEINE IN MILLIGRAMS
Brewed coffee—one cup (5 ounces)	100–150
Instant coffee—one cup	85–100
Decaffeinated coffee—one cup	2–4
Tea—one cup	60–75
Cocoa—one cup	40–55
Chocolate bar	25
Cola—8 ounces	40–60
Anacin	32
Bromo seltzer	32
Cope	32
Darvon Compound	32
Excedrin	65
Midol	32
Pre-mens	30
Vanquish	33

remedies. So we're used to associating it with recreational beverages or, sometimes, with medication.

Nevertheless, caffeine has a potent effect on our bodies. When used properly, it helps relieve headache, but it may have a particularly troubling effect if it is overused.

HOW CAFFEINE CAUSES HEADACHES

Caffeine is a stimulant, which means it stimulates many organs and glands of the body to extra effort. In that way, it is like any other type of emotional or physical stressor, signaling the body to marshal its resources for "fight or flight." As we've seen in Chapter 2, this bodily response may trigger headaches, particularly if there is no physical release for the pent-up energy that is generated.

Exactly how does this process work? Apparently, caffeine stimulates your adrenal glands, the part of the body charged with mobilizing your response to an emergency. The adrenal glands produce adrenaline, which is the signal for your liver to convert its stored-up energy, glycogen, back into glucose or blood sugar. If you take sugar in your coffee, tea, or soda, your blood now has two additional sources of blood sugar—the processed sugar, and the newly converted glucose.

All of this sugar in your blood stimulates your pancreas to produce huge amounts of insulin, which in turn stimulates your adrenal glands a second time. The adrenaline that these glands produce constricts the blood vessels, so that blood can travel through them with more force.

After the constriction, of course, comes the opposite reaction: dilation. Now too much blood is flowing through your arteries, producing the feeling of a throbbing pain that we experience as headache.

Most people don't get headaches when they're "high" on caffeine, only when the effects of the caffeine wear off. That's because for these people, the caffeine has the effect of keeping their blood vessels constricted. Thus, missing a cup of coffee at the usual time may induce your blood vessels to dilate—setting the headache process in motion once again. This is called a caffeine rebound headache due to caffeine withdrawal.

You might think, then, that the solution to caffeine-related headaches is simply to keep your body perpetually stimulated by caffeine. Unfortunately, this is not a good solution. First, in order for this to work, you'd have to perpetually increase your dosage of caffeine, as your body would continually adapt to the lower levels. Secondly, caffeine has a host of other side effects, which increase dramatically as your caffeine intake goes up.

CAFFEINE AND ITS EFFECTS

After swallowing about one gram of caffeine—about eight or ten cups of coffee—your body's reactions include rapid breathing, rapid heartbeat and palpitations, restlessness and excitement, increased urination, insomnia, as well as the more dramatic symptoms of ringing in the ears and disturbances of vision.

Even a more "normal" caffeine intake produces both mood and sleep disturbances, plus lightheadedness and palpitations. People may also experience muscle twitching and gastrointestinal distress.

Sleep disturbances include having trouble falling asleep at night and waking up during the night for no apparent reason. If you are also taking sleeping pills or tranquilizers, caffeine combats their effect, possibly causing you to take increased amounts of those powerful drugs.

Then, after the high of excess stimulation comes the crash of excess fatigue. People experience both physical exhaustion or drowsiness and an emotional letdown or depression when the effects of the caffeine wear off, leading coffee, tea, and cola drinkers to continue their habits even if they're aware of the unpleasant side effects. These include grogginess, drowsiness, lethargy, irritability, and depression, as well as yawning, running nose, headache, and possibly nausea.

One famous study of patients experiencing symptoms of anxiety, insomnia, and dizziness found that rather than the original diagnosis of "anxiety neurosis," these people were suffering from caffeine intoxication. Once they restricted their intake of caffeine, they improved dramatically.

How Much Is Too Much?

For most people, 300 to 400 milligrams of caffeine—three to four cups of brewed coffee—is too much. To find that limit for other forms of caffeine, see Table 7.1 on page 205.

If you're a habitual coffee, tea, or cola drinker, you may not be aware of the strain you're putting on your system, since your body tends to adapt. Complete withdrawal from caffeine for at least three weeks is necessary to experience what a decaffeinated life is like. People who have tried this have reported sleeping much more deeply, experiencing greater vigor, and a sharp decline in headaches, even though they were not aware of sleep or energy problems before cutting back on caffeine.

If you are drinking large amounts of caffeine during the day, you may tend to suffer withdrawal at night, while you sleep. Hence the syndrome of waking up each morning with a headache. Your response is probably to drink more coffee—and possibly to take some caffeine-containing Anacin or Excedrin to "cure" the headache, as well. If caffeine really is the source of the problem, that's like a heroin addict "curing" withdrawal symptoms by taking another shot.

We recommend giving up caffeine completely for three to four weeks, just to become aware of the effect it's having on your body. You may experience additional headaches, drowsiness, irritability, and other withdrawal symptoms, but these should disappear within two weeks at the most. It's possible to avoid or at least reduce these symptoms by tapering off your use of caffeine gradually, cutting back a half-cup or a cup at a time at four- to five-day intervals over a three-week period.

After your first caffeine-free month, you may be amazed at the sense of well-being you experience—a sense that, while drinking caffeine, you're not even aware of missing!

If you still wish to drink some caffeinated beverages after your month-long experiment, keep yourself down to one or two cups (not mugs!) of coffee per day, or the equivalent in other forms of caffeine (see Table 7.1).

WEEKEND HEADACHES AND CAFFEINE

As we've said, if you sleep late on weekends, your body may be going into withdrawal due to being deprived of your regular eight o'clock coffee. Some people drink regular coffee at work and decaffeinated coffee on the weekend, which can also cause rebound headache (the headache you get when deprived of a substance that affects blood vessel activity). (For more on "weekend headaches," see Chapter 2, as well as the section on hypoglycemia, above.)

WHAT ABOUT DECAF?

Unfortunately, decaffeinated coffee, while low in caffeine, does contain some of the chemicals that were used to remove the caffeine. This is true even of water-processed decaf: Although water is used to wash the coffee beans, another chemical is used to draw the caffeine out into the water. Some of the decaffeinating chemicals in the various processes have been shown to cause cancer in animals used in lab experiments. The final word on the safety of these beverages is not yet in.

HEADACHES AND ALCOHOL

As you can see, there's a lot of debate about which substances are related to headache and why. The one thing almost everyone agrees on, however, is that people who are prone to headaches should avoid alcohol. Alcohol, particularly red wine and brandy, is one of the most reliable headache triggers there is.

HOW ALCOHOL CAUSES HEADACHES

Like many of our other headache triggers, alcohol works to dilate the blood vessels. It has a strong hypoglycemic effect, signaling the pancreas that there is an excess of sugar in the blood. If you have a tendency to hypoglycemia anyway, drinking will provoke a vast excess of insulin production, causing your blood sugar level to drop far below normal. This in turn is likely to provoke a headache.

For a fuller explanation of this process, see the above section on headaches and hypoglycemia.

But liquor's effects on blood sugar are only one of the many ways in which this otherwise pleasant substance works to give us headaches. Many liquors contain tyramine and histamine, which, as explained in the above section on amines, are also headache triggers with blood vessel–dilating effects.

Alcohol also interferes with water retention by inhibiting ADH, a pituitary hormone that works to conserve water. Thus drinking can lead to increased urination and then to dehydration. In longtime drinkers, dehydration becomes a serious long-term problem. But even one night of drinking can cause dehydration to a slight degree. Your brain floats in a pool of liquid that keeps it stable and protected within your skull. Dehydration affects this pool of liquid, the temporary depletion of which causes hangover headaches even in people who are normally *not* headache-prone. Dehydration also affects nerve cells in the brain.

Finally, alcohol contains many *congeners,* the flavor and color elements in the liquors. These congeners are related to both the aging and the flavoring process, so their effect varies from liquor to liquor. Generally, however, the greatest likelihood of headache comes from liquor with the greatest number of congeners. Thus the darkest alcohols—brandy, scotch, bourbon, and red wine—are most likely to produce headaches. The lightest-colored alcohols—gin, vodka, and white wine—are less likely to do so.

ALCOHOL AND YOUR LIVER

Alcohol interferes with the functioning of the liver in a variety of ways, many of which are related to headaches. First, its hypoglycemic effect causes an overproduction of insulin, which in turn causes blood sugar levels to drop drastically. This in turn strains the liver, which must convert some stored energy, or glycogen, back into blood sugar, or glucose. In addition, alcohol contains many toxins, which the liver must work overtime to absorb.

DRINKING PATTERNS AND HEADACHES

Only you can decide which drinking patterns are right for you. It's possible that total abstention is the only realistic way to prevent or reduce your headache pain. It's also possible that a drink will set off a headache under some conditions and not others, or that some types of alcohol trigger headaches in you while others are less likely to do so. Increased body awareness and sensitivity to all the factors that affect your headaches can help you make informed decisions about your drinking.

Meanwhile, here is some additional information that may help you decide more effectively:

The alcoholic beverages with the strongest hypoglycemic effect are the ones that are most concentrated: bourbon, brandy, cognac, gin, rye, scotch, vodka, and whiskey are about 35 to 45 percent alcohol. However, although these drinks have a strong effect on your blood sugar, they actually contain no sugar themselves.

Sweet wines and liqueurs, on the other hand, have an especially high concentration of sugar, which is also likely to provoke a hypoglycemic headache. Even though their alcohol content is only about 15 to 20 percent, their combination of alcohol and sugar is a potent headache trigger.

Beer and ale have no sugar, and are only about 5 percent alcohol. However, these drinks contain maltose, which is a bad carbohydrate for those with hypoglycemic tendencies.

If you must take an occasional drink, your best bet is probably a dry white wine. This beverage has only about 10 to 13 percent alcohol content and contains little or no sugar. Red wines are rich in congeners and tyramine, which bring on headaches.

Drinking on an empty stomach, like eating sugar on an empty stomach, will have the most powerful hypoglycemic effect. Eating some protein and carbohydrates, along with a little fat, prior to drinking, mitigates the effect of the alcohol by delaying the rate at which it's absorbed. (You also won't *feel* so drunk, although the actual effect on your reflexes and ability to drive will be the same.) Thus wine with dinner, or a drink with some cheese and crackers is less likely to set off a headache.

At the end of an evening when you've had something to drink, make sure you drink several glasses of water before going to bed. This combats alcohol's dehydrating effect. You might also want to take some vitamin C and one or two aspirins, to combat the effects of a hangover in advance. When you wake up the next morning, drink some more glasses of water and some fruit juice, to raise your blood sugar levels gently but effectively. Do *not* drink more alcohol; this will almost certainly worsen the slight headache you may already have.

VITAMINS AND HEADACHES

There's a lot of controversy over the proper role of vitamins in a healthy diet. We personally believe that while the healthy diet *should* contain all the necessary vitamins, most people simply don't pay close enough attention to such balance, nor do they always have access to enough fresh fruits, grains, and vegetables. Therefore, vitamin supplements may be helpful in some cases.

Vitamin B

The most helpful vitamin for headache sufferers is probably vitamin B. Indeed, there's some evidence that people with migraines have a lifelong deficiency of some forms of this vitamin. Little wonder, since caffeine, birth control pills, alcohol, and stress all tend to destroy vitamin B!

In addition to helping the body cope with stress, vitamin B aids the intermediary metabolism—the digestion and transformation of food on the molecular level. It particularly helps with the metabolism of sugar and carbohydrates, which is why it may help people with hypoglycemic tendencies.

Niacin

Niacin is a B vitamin that has a direct impact on circulation. Niacin is a part of all living cells, so it's likely to be in your diet anyway. Taking 50 mg of niacin, however, produces the so-called "niacin flush" which some people find helps avert a headache, particularly one triggered by stress.

In some people, however, niacin can also trigger a headache by dilating blood vessels.

Vitamin B₆

We recommend an extra 50–100 mg per day of vitamin B₆ to our headache patients. We do find B₆ a helpful counter to premenstrual syndrome (PMS), and we increase the dose at that time of the month. However, don't take more than 150 mg per day of this vitamin as it can cause nerve dysfunction in those quantities. Broccoli, green peas, potatoes, tomato juice, beef, chicken, and ham are good sources of vitamin B.

Vitamin A

Many people find vitamin A supplements to have beneficial effects on their skin, eyes, sinuses, and general health. However, high doses of vitamin A can trigger headaches in people who are headache prone. Normal individuals who take an excess of vitamin A may develop a serious illness called *pseudotumor cerebri,* whose symptoms include headaches, double vision, and increased pressure in the brain. The combination of Vitamin A and tetracycline taken for acne may cause this condition.

Vitamin A is found in bran flakes, cantaloupe, broccoli, carrots, spinach, and turnips.

We recently discharged a sixteen-year-old high school girl from the Greenwich Hospital headache unit after a frightening bout of severe headaches which turned out to be related to her use of vitamins and medication. She had a history of migraine *prior* to developing these "new" headaches.

She had been taking the antibiotic tetracycline plus vitamin A for acne for almost one year. Her dermatologist had been raising her dose of the antibiotic because she was not responding. She began to get severe pains in the front of her head and she thought her vision was slightly blurred. In spite of taking three strong medicines for her headache, she ended up in the emergency room with severe pain.

Her condition was so debilitated that she could not even sit up during her examination and remained lying on

214 / headache relief

the table. Visual testing revealed that the normal blind spot was enlarged in the left eye and she had evidence of increased pressure in the brain as well as swelling of the optic nerve accompanied by small hemorrhages in the retina.

She was admitted to the hospital for an emergency CAT scan of the brain which was entirely normal. A spinal tap was done and the pressure of the spinal fluid was 310 (the highest permissible pressure is 200 millimeters of water). With all other tests being normal, the diagnosis was *pseudotumor cerebri*, or increased pressure in the brain caused by a lack or drainage of spinal fluid related to a reaction from tetracycline and vitamin A. The treatment is to stop the offending medications and to give two medicines, one of which reduces the edema or swelling of the brain and one of which decreases the formation of spinal fluid temporarily. In four days she was much improved and in seven days she left the hospital on two different medicines and without headaches.

Foods, vitamins, and prescription medicines can be the triggers for headaches at times, and the headache specialist has to know everything that a patient is taking to make an accurate diagnosis and prescribe the appropriate treatment.

[8]

HEADACHES
AND THE FEMALE CYCLE

IS ANATOMY DESTINY?
A BIOLOGICAL EXPLANATION

IN CHILDHOOD, migraine sufferers are more likely to be male than female. After puberty, however, women with migraine outnumber their male counterparts by almost three to one. One study shows that from 25 to 29 percent of all women get at least one migraine some time in their lives. Another study, conducted in Denmark, found that approximately 20 percent of all women had had at least one migraine by the time they reached middle age. Of course, many women experience daily headache or several migraine attacks per month.

One reason women seem more susceptible to migraine has to do with the body's response to varying estrogen and progesterone levels. Women experience this variation frequently throughout their lives: at menarche (the time menstruation first begins, usually around age twelve to thirteen), at about the time of menstruation itself, during ovulation, or at menopause. Pregnant women or women with total hysterectomies (including the ovaries) also experience radical changes in their estrogen levels.

Interestingly, it may be the change in estrogen levels that triggers or worsens migraine. Migraines seem to be caused by both decreased estrogen (as in the few days before a monthly period, or after menopause or hysterectomy) and increased estrogen (as when women take birth control pills, experience the first trimester of pregnancy, or take hormone replacement therapy for menopause or hysterectomy). This effect seems to vary according to the woman: an estrogen change that produces or worsens one woman's migraine may actually alleviate the migraine of another.

HORMONES AND YOUR LIVER

Hormonal changes also affect a woman's liver, which must break down any excess estrogen or progesterone in her system. A toxic or sluggish liver (such as that found in heavy drinkers, or in those with diets that don't "fit" their systems) will have more trouble handling this extra work.

These breakdowns translate into hormone imbalances —and migraines. As you can see, diet—especially the consumption of alcohol—plays a major role in menstrual migraine. For similar reasons, it also seems to play a significant part in premenstrual syndrome (PMS), as well as in other menstrual discomfort. (For more on the relationship between diet and migraine, see Chapter 7.)

MIGRAINES AND WOMEN

In the rest of this chapter, we'll look at migraines associated with menstruation, pregnancy, the birth control pill, menopause, hysterectomy, and hormone treatments as well as some help that's available for female migraineurs. In addition, we'll look at a type of female headache unrelated to the menstrual cycle, at tension headaches in women, and at women's relationships with their doctors.

Before we proceed, however, we should remind the reader that there also exists a type of headache that is predominantly experienced by men: cluster headaches. It seems that each gender's physiology has its strong points and its weak points, at least when it comes to headaches.

MENSTRUAL MIGRAINES

A thirty-seven-year-old office manager, a mother of two, came to see us with a twenty-four-year history of one or two headaches per month, one of them always starting one or two days prior to her period. The headaches were very severe, one-sided in the temple, sometimes on the right and sometimes on the left. The pain was throbbing, lasting for twelve to twenty-four hours and always associated with nausea, vomiting, and intolerance to light and sound. She had to lie down in a dark room and get someone to watch her children during these episodes. If she was at work she had to be driven home, as she couldn't see clearly. Medications had never helped much and the only time she could remember being without headaches for more than one or two months was during the last six months of each pregnancy. The headaches returned after she stopped breast feeding. Birth control pills had only made her condition worse.

We stopped her birth control pills and placed her on a migraine diet, and gave her small doses of vitamin B_6 daily with increased attention to diet just prior to menses. We gave her Anaprox, an anti-inflammatory medication, starting four days before the projected day of her period. If she did develop a headache, we treated her first with a drug to block her nausea (Phenergan) and then Cafergot (containing ergotamine tartrate) to shrink the dilated blood vessels in the head. On rare occasions she needed a Fiorinal tablet, when the pain became excruciating.

Within two months her menstrual migraine attacks markedly diminished and the ones she did get were tolerable. She started a daily conditioning program, lost fifteen pounds, and sees us only two times per year and is doing very well.

Up to 60 percent of female migraineurs get their headaches just before, during, or just after menstruation. About 14 percent get them only then. If a woman seems to get headaches only around the time of her period, it's likely that she'll have started getting migraines at menarche (the time of one's first period). Women with this migraine pattern are likely to experience fewer migraines during the second two trimesters of pregnancy. It's fairly certain that her migraines are caused by the falling levels of estrogen during pregnancy and while breast feeding.

218 / HEADACHE RELIEF

If this profile fits you, you can make use of the knowledge to pay particular attention to diet, exercise, and stress during the week before your period is due. Don't expect, however, that just because falling estrogen seems to be the cause of your migraine, taking estrogen will prevent headaches. In fact, the opposite is probably true: As we describe below, taking estrogen supplements, whether in birth control pills, after a hysterectomy, or after menopause may not be beneficial for your treatment of migraine. These supplements usually raise your estrogen levels to a point where you may suffer increased migraine—and possible other dangers, as well. Cyclical replacement (that is, twenty-one days on and seven off) is much more likely to increase the frequency of migraine attack than is noncyclical, or daily, hormone replacement. However, a new treatment using estrogen replacement during menses via a skin patch (estradeum patch) may be helpful and safe, according to recent studies in France.

MIGRAINES AND MENARCHE

As we have noted, many women get their first migraine around the time of their first period. Most women begin a pattern of monthly migraines at this time. Some, however, get a prolonged headache that may last for several weeks. This headache is unresponsive to the medications usually used to treat migraines. After many weeks, it stops by itself. Then the cycle of monthly migraines begins.

MENSTRUAL MIGRAINES AND DIET

As we discussed in Chapter 7, many foods are implicated in triggering migraines. These are foods containing tyramine, phenylethylamine, and nitrites, among others. For women with menstrual migraines, these triggers may operate only around the time of their periods, or the week before. If you have menstrual migraines, you might experiment with staying away from the following foods around the time of your period: chocolate, cold cuts, nuts, aged cheese, and salty foods (for a complete list, see pages 197–98 in Chapter 7).

Many studies have linked migraine to hypoglycemia,

suggesting that headaches are more frequently triggered in people who produce excess amounts of insulin. People with this tendency need to be careful to eat regularly, so that the insulin in their systems does not bring their blood sugar below a certain level. They also need to stay away from processed sugar, which stimulates a rush of insulin. Apparently, a high level of insulin production triggers the release of catecholamines, which in turn trigger a migraine. (For a more thorough explanation of this process, see Chapter 7.)

As we describe in Chapter 7, there's a chance that you have a problem with low blood sugar if you find yourself becoming irritable or panicky when you miss a meal, or within an hour or so after you've eaten something sweet. If you have these tendencies, even occasionally, you may want to be especially careful around the time of your period and the week before. Stay away from processed sugar, and be sure to eat small meals of protein and carbohydrates regularly and frequently, possibly up to every two hours. Before going to bed, have a light snack of crackers and possibly some mild cheese, to make sure your blood sugar levels don't fall too low during the night.

You may also want to try staying away from alcohol. In addition to their triggering function for migraine, alcoholic beverages put an additional strain on your liver, by introducing new toxins into your body. Before your premenstrual week, your liver has already had extra work in breaking down the estrogen in your system. Giving it the added difficulty of processing alcohol can be the final burden that triggers a headache.

Finally, many migraineurs find that headaches are triggered by caffeine. The caffeine acts as a vasoconstrictor—that is, it stimulates your blood vessels to narrow down. Then, when the effect of the caffeine wears off, your blood vessels may dilate, setting off the pattern that brings on a migraine. Even if you don't normally have this reaction, you may be more vulnerable to it during the week before your period. If so, you might want to avoid coffees, teas, and soft drinks containing caffeine. (For more information on migraine and diet, see Chapter 7.)

Knowing whether your migraines are related to menstruation gives you a distinct advantage in preventing them. As you increase your body awareness, you will be able to tell more accurately when certain food or drink is likely to set off a headache. You'll learn which items inevitably cause migraines, and which do so only sometimes. You'll learn to recognize the times when these "sometime" triggers will have their greatest effect—most likely, during the week before your period, but possibly at other stressful times, too. The more you know about when and how your headaches begin, the more you can work in partnership with your body to prevent their pain.

PREGNANCY

Most women who have migraines report some increased headache pain in the first trimester. This is especially troubling since most migraine medication should not be taken during pregnancy. The good news is that over 70 percent of women with migraines report a marked alleviation of migraines during the second and third trimesters of pregnancy—sometimes the only headache improvement they have known during their entire adult lives.

One possibility for this improvement is that the consistently high estrogen levels of pregnancy help prevent migraine. The improvement might also have something to do with the extra endorphins that our body produces during the later stages of pregnancy. Endorphins are morphine-like substances produced by the brain that create a feeling of euphoria and pleasure. Many women, with and without migraines, report euphoric feelings during the later months of their pregnancy. Endorphins are also produced during exercise, which is why exercise is so highly recommended both for depression and for people with headaches.

Even if there has been an improvement in headaches during pregnancy, the migraines will probably return when your periods do. In fact, some women continue to experience more difficulties with headaches during pregnancy—and some women get the first or worst migraines of their lives at or soon after delivery. In one study of forty women on a postnatal ward, fifteen of them got headaches in the first week after giving birth, mostly within the first three to six days. There was a higher rate of headache among those who'd had a previous history of migraines, but even women who had never had a migraine in their lives had their first bout at this time.

Just as the consistently high levels of estrogen during pregnancy seem to help prevent migraine, the postpartum fluctuation in estrogen and progesterone levels seems to be the cause for this increased severity and frequency of migraine after pregnancy. One researcher has hypothesized that falling levels of estradiol (one type of estrogen) sensitize blood vessels, making them more vulnerable to the tendency of serotonin to constrict them. As we've seen, blood vessel constriction then sets off a process that results in migraine. (For more on this process, and on the role of serotonin, see Chapter 2.) However, we don't know why this sensitivity is felt by some women and not others.

Another possible hypothesis for why some women develop migraine after pregnancy is that pregnancy and delivery cause alterations in a woman's metabolism of serotonin, another substance produced by the brain and related to the way the body handles stress, pain, and blood vessel constriction. (For more information on serotonin, see Chapter 1.) Much work remains to be done in this area.

Meanwhile, if you are pregnant or considering pregnancy, it's all the more urgent for you to develop drugless ways of treating and preventing your headaches. We feel that occasional Tylenol or Tylenol with codeine can be used during pregnancy. We think that expectant mothers should avoid ergotamines and preventive medications. Attention to diet and exercise, as well as learning relaxation techniques and new ways of coping with stress may offer you the same relief as medication, in addition to being healthier for you and your baby. Many of the substances that migraineurs should avoid—alcohol, caffeine, nicotine, foods high in processed sugar—are also foods that pregnant women should avoid. Your pregnancy may be the occasion for you

222 / HEADACHE RELIEF

to gain a body awareness and develop new habits that will benefit you long after the delivery.

MENOPAUSE

This stage of the female cycle has a varied effect on migraines. Just as each woman's experience of menopause is different, so is each women's experience of its effect on her headaches. The majority of women seem to have more headaches as they go into menopause, as well as during menopause; they seem to have fewer headaches afterwards.

For some women, migraines simply stop after menopause. Apparently, the hormonal factors that once set off migraines are no longer operating in the same way. Likewise, foods, drinks, or stressors that once triggered headaches are now handled differently.

For other women, migraines may become worse. They come more often, or bring more intense pain, or both. Again, much research remains to be done in this field, and we can't yet say what produces this effect, beyond the speculation that it has something to do with hormone levels, which in turn affects the extent to which arteries constrict.

What we can say with assurance is that the kind of body awareness, diet, exercise, and relaxation techniques that we've been recommending can only help the woman experiencing or about to experience menopause. You should avoid alcohol, sugar, and salt. A vigorous but reasonable exercise schedule, as suggested by your doctor, will alleviate stress and produce the endorphins that create a sense of calm and well-being. A person who has learned to listen to her body, to be sensitive to how it reacts to various foods as well as to various life events, will be far better equipped to cope with the chemical changes of menopause. And these chemical changes themselves may be modified by finding the diet and the exercise that is right for you.

For some women, menopause is not a difficult transition to make, either physically or emotionally. For others, menopause is quite difficult, either because of what it seems to symbolize about age, attractiveness, and sexuality, or because of the effects of biochemical changes, or both. In any of these cases, though, a person who has learned relaxation techniques and ways of coping with stress will have within herself additional ways of coping with any difficulties that menopause may bring. And that woman's sense of mastery, of being able to heal herself, will in itself affect the way she faces her new condition—and the way it affects her.

For more information on hormone treatments after menopause, see below.

HYSTERECTOMY

It might seem that if migraines are brought on by menstruation, an operation that ends menstruation would end the migraines. Unfortunately, this doesn't seem to be true. Like menopause, hysterectomy is both an emotional and a physical issue. Both its emotional stressors and its physical effects can increase the likelihood of migraine. Some women do report alleviation of their migraines after total hysterectomy, but the vast majority do not. It is absolutely not recommended as a treatment for migraine.

HORMONE TREATMENTS

Many doctors prescribe estrogen replacement therapy for menopause and hysterectomy. This may further aggravate a woman's migraines, depending on the manner of replacement.

Furthermore, hormone treatments for migraineurs can increase the risk of stroke, heart attack, and cancer. Migraines in any case may be associated with a greater risk of stroke. This risk is increased again if you're a smoker. The combination of smoking, migraines, and hormone treatments is a triple threat.

In our opinion, migraineurs should avoid hormone treatments if at all possible. If medically necessary, you might have better luck with a synthetic estrogen, rather than one made from animal hormones. You should use very low doses of estrogen. The estrogen patch may deliver the hormone in a safe way, with few if any side effects and good migraine relief. The patch is placed on an area of clean, dry skin on the abdomen. It must be changed twice weekly. It delivers small, constant doses of the naturally occuring ovarian hormone 17 beta-estradiol. This may cause fewer headaches than oral preparations given cyclically (twenty-one days on, seven days off).

THE BIRTH CONTROL PILL AND THE MORNING-AFTER PILL

Both of these pills are composed of hormones that affect a woman's menstrual cycle. As with hormone treatments for menopause or hysterectomy, these medications can be both uncomfortable and dangerous for women with migraines.

BIRTH CONTROL PILLS

In most women, birth control pills produce an increased likelihood of migraine, and of headache in general. Most migraineurs who take "the pill" notice that their headaches come more frequently, and with more intensity.

An estimated 50 percent or more of women who have never had migraines before have them after taking the pill. As with menstrual and pregnancy migraines, these headaches seem to be related to fluctuations in hormones. Possibly women who had a tendency in this direction but never actually suffered from migraine are "pushed over the edge" by the new hormone fluctuations on which the pill depends.

If taking the pill does bring on new or increased migraines, it is likely to do so within the first several months, although some women do experience a worsening years later—possibly triggered by some other factor in combination with the strain already produced by the pill. If a woman then stops taking the pill, her headaches are likely to be relieved—but slowly, again, over several months. In some cases, however, the headaches stop immediately, particularly if the woman hasn't been taking the pill for very long.

Occasionally, women do report a lessening of their migraines after they start taking the pill. In either case, however, the pill may increase your risk of stroke, which is already slightly greater than average if you are a migraineur. Particularly if your headaches become worse after taking the pill, the increased risk of stroke is even more likely. Again, the combination of having migraines, taking the pill, and smoking is especially dangerous, greatly upping your risk of stroke, heart attack, and cancer. We never prescribe birth control pills for women with migraine, and we suggest they stop the pill if they are currently taking it.

THE MORNING-AFTER PILL

The morning-after pill (diethylstilbestrol, or DES), taken to discourage a possible pregnancy, is not taken as regularly as birth control pills are, but it too increases your risk of cancer, heart attack, and stroke. Of course, no one should rely on this pill as a means of birth control, but migraineurs least of all. Taking it once or twice after an unplanned sexual encounter may do no more than set off another migraine, but taking it with any degree of regularity is likely to increase both your headaches and your risk.

WHAT YOU CAN DO ABOUT "FEMALE CYCLE" MIGRAINES

There are two things you can do to cope with your "female cycle" migraines. One is to study the suggestions on diet, exercise, and relaxation that we make in the other chapters of this book. The other is to develop your body awareness, especially around the time of your period. You'll be surprised at how much you already know about what foods are likely to set off a headache, or what bodily sensations are really signals warning you to turn down that glass of wine.

Ways of coping with menstrual migraines, particularly, are similar to advice for coping with premenstrual syndrome (PMS). Many migraineurs also suffer from PMS, a not-yet-well-understood combination of symptoms that some women get during the week before their period, including irritability, anxiety, and depression, as well as some physical symptoms that include retention of water and a tendency to headache.

Both migraineurs and women with PMS should pay special attention to their diet during the week before their periods, avoiding salt, sugar, and alcohol. As we've said, migraineurs should also avoid chocolate, aged cheese, cold cuts, and smoked meats.

On the other hand, the week before a period is not the time for a migraineur to miss meals, start a crash diet, or cut back on whole grains, potatoes, or pasta. These high carbohydrate foods are excellent for coping both with stress and with the fluctuations in blood sugar that many studies have associated with migraine. Generally, women with either syndrome would benefit from a diet high in protein and carbohydrates and low in sugar, salt, and fat.

Vitamin Supplements

Vitamin B_6 can be given in doses of 50 to 150 mg per day. This vitamin is also a natural diuretic.

We have also found it helpful for women who are premenstrual to take Vitamin E supplements of 400 IU per day, which is considerably higher than the recommended daily allowance, which is 10 mg. Women with menstrual migraines might also benefit from taking multivitamins. Since the birth control pill tends to deplete the body's supply of vitamin B_6, women who are taking the pill or who have ever taken it may be especially in need of this essential vitamin, which supports the proper functioning of the nervous system. Caffeine also destroys the body's supply of B vitamins.

On the other hand, the so-called megadoses of B vitamins have been known to cause toxicity in some female migraineurs. We recommend that your supplement not exceed the RDA allowance, unless you are working under the supervision of a nutritionist, physician, or other qualified health care practitioner.

As we've already noted, exercise is extremely useful in preventing female cycle migraines. It improves the circulation, which, as we know, is disrupted by the migraine process. It also helps the brain to produce endorphins, which have both physical and psychological benefits.

FEMALE CYCLE MIGRAINES AND MEDICATION

Most medication used for the prevention or treatment of migraines can't be used during pregnancy, because of their dramatic impact on the fetus. We rarely permit, except in extreme circumstances, medication during pregnancy. However, we do prescribe some combination of preventive and symptomatic medication to women with menstrual migraines, when they are not pregnant, during menopause, or after total hysterectomy.

Some nonsteroidal anti-inflammatory drugs have been found to be useful for women with hormonally related migraines. Bellergal and other related drugs may help prevent such migraines, as can ergotamine tartrate. (For more information on these drugs and their side effects, see Chapter 3.) The estrogen patch as mentioned above can be helpful in menstrual migraine.

"BAD" HEADACHES: ANOTHER KIND OF FEMALE HEADACHE

There is another kind of "woman's" headache, one that is *not* related to hormonal fluctuations. Doctors have named it the "benign autonomic dysfunction" (or BAD) headache.

This headache comes from a benign (non-life-threatening) heart defect known as the "mitral valve prolapse." In this defect, one of the doors (valves) to a heart chamber doesn't close completely. The headache related to this condition is accompanied by chest pain and a speeded-up heartbeat. It may also be accompanied by changes in blood pressure, or some emotional disturbances.

Women who are susceptible to this type of headache

may notice that they get flushed, or break out in red blotches on their chest and neck when they are irritated or excited. They may also have larger pupils than normal.

Because this condition is in no way a threat to life or an indicator of heart disease, it hasn't received much attention, but as many as 10 percent of all women may have it, for a total of 14 or 15 million women. The percentage of female migraineurs who experience this condition is even higher: some 15 to 20 percent.

Drugless treatments for this condition are essentially the same as the others we've discussed in this chapter. Medical treatments may include prescribing propranolol HCl (Inderal) or some other beta blocker.

WOMEN AND TENSION

Although we have said repeatedly that there is no such thing as a "headache personality," there are some psychological patterns that can trigger headaches, of both the migraine and the muscle contraction variety. This doesn't mean that women with either type of headache are more likely to experience such patterns than other women; only that their way of reacting to these emotional issues is likely to result in a headache.

One of the strongest psychological triggers for a headache of any type is unexpressed anger. In our culture, women tend to have a harder time expressing their anger than men do. Many women are brought up to believe that it isn't "feminine" to get mad, and that it's certainly not ladylike to let your anger show.

Or a woman may feel that, regardless of her own feelings about it, her anger is likely to be misunderstood by those around her, or that she will be treated badly as a result of expressing her rage. A woman who loses her temper with a coworker who makes a patronizing or sexually suggestive remark, for example, may feel that other coworkers will interpret her anger as evidence that she can't handle the pressures of the job, or that she can't take the normal round of workplace joking.

Women who are in nontraditional positions, either because of the type of job they are working at or because of the high level of their position at work, may feel under even greater pressure to control their feelings, particularly those of anger. They may feel that expressing anger either at work or at home will be interpreted as evidence that they have taken on "too much" and should therefore "do less," that is, give up the position they've achieved.

Suggesting solutions for these underlying problems is, of course, beyond the scope of this book. But, if you are a woman who regularly suffers from any type of headache, we do suggest that you consider the possibility that you're suppressing some powerful emotions, especially anger. If there's even a slight chance that this may be the case, ask yourself which will be more painful: continuing to have your headaches, or undergoing a process of learning more about yourself and these emotions. This process might include some form of psychotherapy or counseling, or you may prefer to focus on some other method of coping, such as meditation, biofeedback training, or relaxation techniques.

Many women, particularly those who are working at high-pressure jobs or who are working both inside and outside the home, are worried about looking into this area. They may feel that they have to defend themselves against the pressures to "do less"—that is, to aim lower, to take fewer risks. Or they may feel that if they really looked at their feelings, they would be "forced" to give up some of their activities or relationships.

It's possible that your self-exploration will lead you to make some changes in your life. It's also possible that therapy or meditation will lead you to increase your work activities and improve your existing relationships. Either way, if you are regularly experiencing disabling headaches, you are already facing a serious obstacle to your productivity and your relationships with others. Uncovering suppressed emotions and dealing with them may ultimately be a better choice for you.

Once again, we are *not* suggesting that your headaches are "all psychological." We are suggesting that your emo-

tions are one important component of your life. Along with
diet, exercise, hormones, and a host of other factors, they
too affect your body and deserve your attention.

WOMEN AND DOCTORS

Unfortunately, the syndrome we described in Chapter
1, in which doctors fail to take headaches seriously, prescribe inappropriate medication for them, or overmedicate
without regard to side effects, is even more likely to happen
to women patients. Our culture often tends to disregard
women's feelings and experiences, or to believe women
less reliable observers than men. Doctors are no less a part
of the culture than anyone else. Thus women patients may
sometimes feel that their doctors are not taking them seriously.

As we've said, many doctors are already prone to prescribing symptomatic treatment (painkillers or tranquilizers) for headache, rather than to search for a solution that
deals with a headache's causes. This tendency is especially
present with female patients. Even when they are not dealing with headache patients, doctors seem to have a tendency to overprescribe for women. Thus Valium, a
powerfully addictive tranquilizer, has been one of the most
overprescribed drugs in the United States and one of the
most abused—almost entirely because doctors have inap-
propriately prescribed it for women. A doctor who thinks
that his female patient simply needs a pill to help her "calm
down" is neither likely to work with you to determine
which diet and exercise patterns are most helpful for you,
nor to help you explore therapies and relaxation techniques.

Such a doctor is also unlikely to work with you to determine whether this particular drug or dosage is right for
you. Such a doctor may not sufficiently explain the side
effects you should watch out for, or may not schedule frequent enough visits to monitor your progress. He or she
may not be aware of the analgesic rebound effect, in which,
the more painkillers you take, the worse your headaches

become. Instead, as your headache pills become less effective, such a doctor may simply continue to increase your dosage or prescribe a stronger medication.

Likewise, if your medication produces a side effect, such a doctor may simply prescribe some additional medication to combat the effect. This in turn may create a new effect, which in turn is medicated with a new drug, setting up a painful and debilitating cycle of disorders, medication, and side effects.

In one extreme example—though one which rarely happens—a woman with migraines may be prescribed ergotamine to prevent the headaches' occurrence. The ergotamine aggravates her tendency to hypertension, so she is given a beta blocker (propranolol HCl or Inderal) to combat her high blood pressure. This raises her cholesterol level, so she is put on an anti-cholesterol diet that actually aggravates her migraines. Furthermore, the drugs she is taking increase her tendency to gain weight, which further increases her blood pressure. The drugs and her inability to control her headaches and her weight contribute to her depression, so she is given tranquilizers. The tranquilizers cause her to become slightly disoriented and less effective in her decision-making abilities, which further worsens her depression. And so on.

As doctors ourselves, we're certainly not making a wholesale condemnation of the medical profession. Nor are we condemning medication, which has been an effective, safe, and satisfying course of treatment for many of our patients. We use medication frequently, but appropriately, and with good education for the patient as to how to take it, possible side effects, and when to call us. In this spirit, we encourage you to take full responsibility for your choice of doctor, so that you find yourself working with a health care professional who respects you and deserves your trust.

Your trust and cooperation are important to both you and your physician. The search for headache treatment may be long and painful. It may require some trial and error, or you may have to endure some temporary pain. If you need to withdraw from analgesics, for example, you may experience enormous difficulty before benefiting from considerable relief. This process is difficult, but can be made easier by a compassionate professional whom you trust to know the difference between necessary and unnecessary pain.

Every human body is unique, with its own set of chemical and emotional reactions. A medication and dosage that produce horrific side effects in one person may seem like a miracle cure to another. It's important that you and your doctor establish a partnership to explore the treatment that is best for you, so that you fully cooperate in the search for your proper treatment. Without your accurate reports on your condition, the professional working with you can't know what's working and what isn't.

On page 43 in Chapter 1, we've provided a brief checklist of questions to ask yourself about your current health care practitioner. If answering these questions provokes you to be dissatisfied with your doctor, discuss your concerns with him or her. If you still feel dissatisfied, perhaps you should begin the search for a new practitioner. Ask these questions of the new professionals you are considering, until you're satisfied that you've found someone who deserves your respect and trust. Then give that person your full cooperation, and take full responsibility for your own part in healing yourself.

[9]

THE LITTLEST VICTIMS:
CHILDREN AND HEADACHES

CHILDHOOD HEADACHES:
A FAMILY CONCERN

YOU LOOK AT your child curled up in bed, looking pale and sick. You see the pain, and you feel helpless, perhaps even guilty. Is this something you caused? Is it somehow your fault? Why can't you do anything to make it go away? Your child's eyes are closed as he or she tries to sleep, but the pain won't permit it. You don't like the idea of your son or daughter being on medication at such a young age, but this is the third day this week that the child hasn't gone to school. Your other children are starting to feel that the sick one gets all the attention, and you're concerned about this, too. Is there anything you can do?

Fortunately, there is. Childhood headache is a difficult disorder, not only for your child, but for the entire family. But just as the entire family is affected by one child's headache, the entire family can participate in helping the child to get well.

In this chapter, we'll look at the types of childhood headache that are most common, distinguishing between those that are the result of some other condition and those that are "just headaches." We'll suggest some ways of working effectively with your child's health care practitioner, and review the various medications that may be prescribed in extreme cases. We'll look at the drugless types of treatment that are available for your child. And we'll review some ways that you and the other members of your family can support your child's coping with headache.

As you read this chapter, take heart. The prognosis for your child is very good. Boys, especially, often outgrow their childhood migraines. Some one-third of all children grow out of their headache patterns completely, with 15 percent suddenly becoming headache-free each year. Even those children whose headaches don't simply disappear can be greatly helped by the diet and behavioral approaches described in this chapter. And the skills that your child learns in the process will be a lifelong source of strength and self-reliance.

HOW COMMON ARE CHILDHOOD HEADACHES?

The answer is: very common. Because there are so few studies, and because definitions of different types of headache vary so widely, it's difficult to cite statistics with any sense of certainty. But the figures that are available certainly indicate that many children have headaches, some from a very early age, indeed.

We do know that about one-quarter of all adult migraineurs suffered in childhood, as well. And over half of the adults who will have migraine have had at least one attack by age twenty. In 70 to 90 percent of these cases, there is a family history of migraine, sometimes on both the father's and the mother's side.

One famous study found that 40 percent of the children studied had had some kind of headache before the age of seven, while by fifteen, 75 percent had had one. Another study suggested that 20 percent of all seven year olds have one or more headaches per month. By age fourteen, 70 percent of the children studied had had at least one headache, with 30 percent having them at least once a month.

Migraines have been reported in children as young as twelve to eighteen months. The early age of six seems to be the average time for migraine attacks to begin. One study showed that by age fifteen, 5.3 percent of the children studied were suffering from migraine, with 15.7 percent having frequent nonmigraine headaches and 54 percent having occasional nonmigraine headaches. Another study suggests that the proportion of children with migraine is closer to 10 percent.

We can summarize these sometimes conflicting data by saying that by age fifteen, we believe that some 75 to 82 percent of all children have had some kind of headache, with 7 to 18 percent of them suffering from migraine. About 60 percent of these child migraineurs are male, although the proportion starts to reverse in adolescence when girls are getting their periods, and, frequently, their first migraines as well. (For more on the association between migraine and the beginning of menstruation, see Chapter 8.) After puberty, the ratio goes from 60/40 percent to 30/70 percent, which is the eventual ratio of male to female migraineurs.

WHAT KIND OF HEADACHE DOES YOUR CHILD HAVE?

Approximately 5 percent of children with chronic, recurring headaches are suffering from serious illness or a medical/neurological problem, rather than migraine or muscle contraction headache. Almost invariably in these cases, other symptoms are present in addition to the headache.

Although these headaches are rare, many parents are concerned about them. Your doctor should make the final diagnosis, but, to help set your mind at ease, we present here some childhood headaches that are *not* migraines, muscle contraction headaches, or cluster headaches. As you can see, few of them are serious conditions, and those that are serious are extremely rare. Thus, whatever their source, it's unlikely that your child's headaches are life-threatening or that they're indicators of any permanently debilitating disease.

SINUS HEADACHES

In our opinion, far too many headaches are attributed to sinusitis, which is actually a relatively rare cause of headache. Perhaps 13 percent of those who have sinusitis may experience headache in the forehead, especially in the area between the eyes. These headaches are almost invariably accompanied by other symptoms: coughing, nasal congestion, runny nose, postnasal drip, ear infections, and apparent "allergic" reactions.

Sinus x-rays often show a thickening of the sinuses' mucous linings. Treatment usually involves antibiotics for acute infections and decongestants for chronic sinusitis, as well as a dairy-free diet to prevent the production of mucus.

However, as we've said, many people come to us believing that their children's headaches are sinus headaches, whereas even when the sinus problem is cleared up, the headache remains. These headaches more often prove to be migraine or muscle contraction headaches.

HEADACHES RELATED TO VISION

Again, these headaches are often misunderstood. People tend to think that squinting, astigmatism, or other eye problems are the cause of headaches, but they rarely are. Sometimes a child will get headache pain across the forehead as a result of watching television, doing schoolwork, or some other extensive use of the eyes. Therefore, these headaches usually occur in the afternoon, after the eyes have been "overworked." If your child is waking up with headaches, or getting them during the morning, it's unlikely that his or her eyes are involved. Sometimes a checkup with an ophthalmologist (eye doctor) is reassuring.

DENTAL HEADACHES

This is still a controversial area: No one can agree on whether dental problems are a common cause of headache or not. Those who do believe that many headaches have dental causes look to the temporomandibular joint, the joint formed between the upper part of the jaw and the temporal bone of the skull. If this joint isn't properly aligned, muscles inside and outside the jaw may contract too much or too tightly, which many believe causes muscle contraction headaches. They offer as evidence the fact that a headache sufferer may feel pain in the joints of the jaw, which is increased by chewing, and that the jaw may not have an adequate range of motion. Most headache experts, however, believe that this is rarely a cause of headache, especially in children.

THE "ICE CREAM HEADACHE"

Some children who are prone to migraine are also likely to get "ice cream" headaches: an intense pain experienced as being behind the eye, or deep behind the bridge of the nose, resulting from eating ice cream or some other cold food too quickly. Apparently, the cold induces a type of neuralgia (pain in the nerves), and a vascular reaction (that is, a problem with blood flow, related to migraine). There's no cause for concern: Simply have the child give the cold treat some time to warm up, and make sure that it is eaten somewhat more slowly.

HIGH FEVER OR INFECTION

If a child has a high fever, headache will often be a "side effect." If this is the only time your child has a headache, your concern should probably be about the cause of the fever, rather than the headache. High fevers and related headaches are frequently associated with flu and other common childhood complaints.

Sometimes an infectious disease may cause a child's headache. *Meningitis* is caused by a skull fracture, a penetrating wound, or the spread of another infection into the brain. *Tuberculous meningitis* is a complication arising from tuberculosis. Both diseases are accompanied by nausea, vomiting, fever, stiff neck, general ill health, lassitude, loss of appetite, and weight loss, as well as by a headache.

Encephalitis, generalized viral infections, and *ear infections* may also be accompanied by headache. Again, these diseases usually have distinctive symptoms. Encephalitis usually follows a mosquito bite in the summer; it causes confusion, hallucinations, sleepiness, epilepsy, and fever. A generalized viral infection is heralded by aches and pains all over, cold-type symptoms, and possible stomach cramps and diarrhea, as well as the headache. An ear infection causes ear pain, sore throat, and decreased hearing on one side.

TUMORS
Many people worry that frequent or recurring headaches are the sign of a brain tumor. This condition is extremely rare, and a headache is almost never the first sign of it. In children under the age of ten, perhaps five in 100,000 will suffer from a brain tumor.

The first symptoms of this condition in children are restlessness, frequent vomiting, crying, irritability, daily headaches, and an increase in pain caused by coughing, sneezing, or other strain. The headaches associated with tumors will change in character, will begin to happen more frequently, or will become more severe, often waking the child from sleep (as opposed to the child waking up in the morning with a headache). The associated vomiting will be persistent, and will often become progressively more frequent.

It's true that some of these symptoms do resemble the signs of childhood migraine, particularly the association of vomiting with the headache. Your doctor should be able to set your mind at ease about this rare condition, so that you can focus on the much more likely reality of your child's having migraines or muscle contraction headaches. Sometimes a CAT scan or MRI (magnetic resonance imaging) scan and an EEG (electroencephalogram) may be ordered.

POSTTRAUMATIC HEADACHES
A posttraumatic headache is a pain that follows a trauma, in this case, a blow to the head or a neck injury. Such a headache is most often located in the specific area where the blow occurred, and it usually ends by itself.

There are two types of posttraumatic headaches:

A *localized pain* isn't accompanied by other symptoms. The headache pain reflects nerve and tissue injury in the area that was struck. Such a pain may last for months, but eventually it goes away without treatment.

Post–concussion syndrome, or *post–head trauma syndrome*, on the other hand, is more serious. It's accompanied by other symptoms: amnesia about the accident, restlessness or lassitude, personality changes, depression, irritability, ongoing memory problems, dizziness, and possibly problems in school. Such a syndrome is hard to treat, but in time, with regular attention, reassurance to the child, and an avoidance of narcotic painkillers, the child can recover. Children with such a syndrome should be regularly examined by a professional.

Children may not remember or be able to tell you about the head injury that may have produced these headaches, particularly if the children are very young. If your child shows signs of headaches of this type, it's helpful to your doctor if you look for evidence of a possible physical injury.

MIGRAINES AND MUSCLE CONTRACTION HEADACHES

IDENTIFYING THE HEADACHE TYPE

If your child suffers regularly from headaches, it's far more likely that he or she has a childhood version of these "adult" headache syndromes, rather than one of the relatively rare conditions described in the preceding section. More information on all of these headache types is available in Chapter 2. Here, we deal specifically with the childhood versions of them.

As we explained in Chapter 2, we like the idea of a continuum among migraines and muscle contraction headaches, because it explains why so many people, adults as well as children, suffer from both types of headaches, and why headaches may switch from one type to another. It also explains why biofeedback, relaxation techniques, dietary changes, and exercise may be similarly beneficial to both types of headache people.

However, even if various headache disorders are related, there are some identifiable syndromes that can be discussed separately. For convenience' sake, we'll continue to talk about migraines and muscle contraction headaches as separate entities, even though the two conditions may be fundamentally related.*

MIGRAINE IN CHILDREN

One of the most painful headache syndromes is migraine. If your child has migraine, chances are excellent that it isn't your first contact with this syndrome: as we've noted, 70 to 90 percent of all children with migraine have a family history of this disease. (Even if you think there's no migraine in your family, you may have misidentified migraines as other types of headaches.)

The word migraine is derived from the Greek word *hemikrania,* which means "half of the head," because many migraineurs experience pain on only one side. In children, however, the pain is frequently felt on both sides. Like adult migraine pain, children's migraines are usually experienced as a throbbing sensation, although pressure and squeezing sensations are reported as well.

Migraine in children generally occurs with greater frequency than in adults. Most child migraineurs get headaches once a week, but some experience headaches several times a week.

A child's migraine can also develop much more rapidly than an adult's, becoming severe in less than an hour. The good news is that children's attacks are generally shorter than those in adults, sometimes lasting as briefly as thirty minutes, although some childhood migraines have been known to continue for several days. Usually, however, the child migraineur will seek a dark, quiet place and fall into a deep sleep for a while. When the child awakens, the headache is usually gone, and color has returned to the child's face.

Children's migraines are usually accompanied by the same symptoms that adults experience, along with some that are unique to childhood. Like adults, children nearly always experience nausea and sensitivity to light during

* For more information on cluster headaches, see Chapter 2. For more information on cluster headaches in children, see below.

their headaches. In addition, children may also feel abdominal pain and listlessness, and may run a fever, sometimes up to 104 degrees Fahrenheit.

Children with migraine almost always experience severe gastrointestinal distress, usually accompanied by vomiting. Sometimes the nausea and vomiting are worse than the headache itself.

Some child migraineurs experience stuffing of the nostrils, rapid heartbeat, dizziness, and the appearance of being very ill. With severe attacks, the child loses all appetite and is sluggish and irritable. Children too young to talk about their pain are irritable, agitated, and crying.

Migraine Triggers

A child's migraine may come before or after a tense or exciting event, such as a school exam, a sporting event, a birthday party, or a family trip. In Britain, some migraines are known as "happy days headaches," since they're triggered by pleasant events as well as by difficult ones.

Diet also plays a key role in children's migraines. Like many adults, child migraineurs may react with headaches to processed sugar or junk food. Likewise, children may get headaches from missing meals or from waiting too long for a meal. If your child's headaches seem to be triggered by sweet foods or missed meals, see Chapter 7 for a fuller discussion of hypoglycemia and migraine.

Children's migraines may be triggered by foods rich in tyramine, such as aged cheeses (including cheddar), liver, yogurt, and bananas; or with a high level of nitrites, such as bacon and smoked meats; chocolate is also a common migraine trigger.

As with adults, stress, fatigue, illness, weather, and traveling in a car or bus may provoke children's migraines. (We'll discuss psychological triggers and behavioral approaches to children's migraines later on.) Some children get migraines from moving into a bright area from a dark one, from steady glare, from the bright light of a sunny day, or from the flickering light of a television or movie screen. Weather changes may bring on a child's migraine, particularly a damp day or a sudden change from dry to damp. A few children get migraines from physical exertion, particularly in such sports as gymnastics, where the head is lower than the rest of the body and also goes through rapid acceleration.

Many girls get their first migraines at the time of their first period, or soon after. We believe that hormonal changes trigger these migraines, which are likely to continue throughout their adult lives. (For more information on migraines and menstruation, see Chapter 8.)

Warning signs for a child's migraine may include the following symptoms on the day before the attack: a heavy head, a lot of yawning, sleepiness, listlessness, or a craving for certain types of foods. These cravings are usually for sweet foods or other migraine triggers, suggesting that blood sugar fluctuations are involved in the child's headaches. If cravings for sweet foods tend to precede your child's migraine, see Chapter 7 for a fuller discussion of migraine and hypoglycemia.

CLASSICAL AND COMMON MIGRAINE

Like adults, children get both of these headache syndromes, with common migraines being more usual than the classical ones. In classical migraine, there are two phases, the aura preceding the headache, and the headache itself. In common migraine without aura, there is only one phase. However, both types of headaches may be preceded by the warning signs described above.

Classical migraine affects about 5 to 10 percent of migraine patients. The aura is the period when the migraineur's intracranial blood vessels (the blood vessels that supply blood to the back of the brain) are constricting, causing a decreased blood flow to the parts of the brain served by those vessels. This produces a type of visual disruption: blind spots, loss of peripheral vision, flickering, colored, zig-zag lines, flashing lights moving across the field of vision, blurring, and so on. In a variation of classical migraine known as "complicated migraine," children experiencing an aura may also develop neurological signs and feel weak on one side of their bodies, experience aphasia (difficulties in speaking or remembering words correctly), or have other sensory distortions, such as numbness, tingling, or loss of feeling (even when they are pricked with pins in a diagnostic test). They may be unable to use one of their limbs, or experience scotoma (holes in their vision), micropsia (objects appearing small), or macropsia (objects appearing large).

In children, the aura usually lasts about twenty or thirty minutes. Sometimes, in both children and adults, the aura is experienced but subsequent headache pain is not. This is known as a migraine equivalent and is a dysfunction of the visual part of the brain, the part in the back or the occipital area, possibly related to decreased blood flow to the visual areas of the brain, as a result of the blood vessels' constriction. Or it may be caused by a dysfunction of the brain cells, triggered by some other biochemical or nervous disorder. In complicated migraine, the parts of the brain that control sensation, vision, and movement may be involved.

In the second phase of all of these types of migraine, the aura disappears, to be replaced by a throbbing pain on one or both sides of the head, usually accompanied by vomiting, abdominal pain, sensitivity to light and sound, and the desire to sleep. In about 20 percent of all child migraineurs, there may be an attack of diarrhea as well. During this phase the child may feel cold and look pale. Usually, the child is finally able to sleep, and the headache is gone when he or she awakes.

The preheadache signs of common migraine are more variable, and may include malaise, personality change, or depression, in place of the clearly defined aura. The actual headache and accompanying symptoms are the same as those of classical migraine.

A nine-year-old boy was brought to us by his parents because he was missing one to two days of school a week. In addition to his absences, he wasn't able to play ball with the other children.

His headaches would start in the late morning or early afternoon, when his stomach began to hurt and he would see brightly colored, blinking wavy lines out of the corner of his eye. These lines would move slowly in front of him,

244 / HEADACHE RELIEF

partially obscuring his vision. They would disappear in twenty to thirty minutes, and he then developed mild to moderate throbbing pain on one side of his head. This pain was accompanied by a generalized cold feeling, nausea, vomiting, and an overwhelming desire to sleep.

This classic childhood migraine was triggered by eating foods with high salt content, or missing a meal for more than two hours, or stress or heavy exercise—or a combination of all of these factors.

He was placed on a program that included a special diet, a regular exercise program, and biofeedback training. After three months, the frequency of his headaches had been reduced from eight or more a week to only two per month. He was also taking one Midrin capsule to control the pain of his remaining, infrequent headaches.

Even though this patient is only nine, he now knows how to avoid his headaches and what to do when he feels one coming on. His case illustrates the important point that the great majority of our patients under the age of fifteen respond well to diet, change in life-style, and biofeedback training or other behavioral techniques. They do not need strong medications that can create possible side effects.

VERTEBROBASILAR MIGRAINE

Another form of childhood migraine is called vertebrobasilar migraine. It's believed to have its origin in the brain stem, the most primitive part of the human brain. It also involves the basilar artery (which supplies blood to the lower brain stem), which is believed to constrict in the pre-headache phase.

Vertebrobasilar migraine is more common in girls than in boys, beginning around the time of their periods and frequently occurring monthly. Like the other forms of childhood migraine, it is likely to occur in children with a strong family history of migraine.

The signs of vertebrobasilar migraine include a loss of equilibrium, disturbed balance, double vision, trouble speaking, slurred speech, confusion, and sometimes even coma or loss of consciousness. The lack of blood in the brain stem, caused by the basilar artery's constriction, produces these symptoms, which indicate neurological involvement.

Sometimes those who suffer from vertebrobasilar headaches simply experience these symptoms, without the headache pain. Fortunately, these headaches tend to resolve themselves by the late teens or early twenties.

OTHER FORMS OF MIGRAINE

There are a few other variants on classical or common migraine that children tend to experience. We imagine that the changes in the child's brain that take place throughout development set off these syndromes, since these versions of migraine are usually not found in adults.

OPHTHALMOPLEGIC MIGRAINE
As the name suggests, these migraines involve dysfunction in the movement of the eye. One of the twelve cranial nerves, often the third or the sixth, may be paralyzed, which causes double vision. The pupil may be enlarged. The child may experience a pain in one eye. The double vision may outlast the headache by days or even weeks.

HEMIPLEGIC MIGRAINE
In this variant, the child experiences paralysis on one side of the body, before the onset of the headaches. The paralysis may be a frightening experience, but it is not permanent. In this type of migraine, the child usually experiences pain on alternate sides of the head with each attack.

MIGRAINE EQUIVALENTS

Another childhood syndrome is known as "migraine equivalents" or sometimes, "migraine variants." This occurs when children experience disturbances in brain and body function that usually accompany some form of migraine, but without the headache pain. They seem to be triggered by some of the same causes of migraine—restricted blood flow, and/or some related neurological disturbance. They're believed to be caused by changes in the brain's activity as the child develops, and many of the symptoms respond to antimigraine therapy, even if there is no headache pain.

Symptoms of migraine equivalents are vertigo (a feeling that the world is spinning, causing imbalance); motion sickness; periodic fainting; seeing flashing or flickering lights; tachycardia (rapid heartbeat); mood disturbances; sleep disturbances; and distortions in the bodily sensations of smell, vision, or body image.

Some migraine equivalents take the form of a state of acute confusion, with disturbed physical sensations and agitation. Bedwetting, night terrors, and sleepwalking may also be caused by a migraine equivalent. These conditions may only later be identified as related to migraine, since they may have other causes.

Sometimes, children aged two to four get a migraine equivalent in the form of episodic vertigo; that is, they periodically feel that the room is spinning and compensate by losing their balance or altering their posture. Sometimes this variant strikes children above the age of four. Generally, this problem resolves itself and no treatment is needed.

The most dramatic symptom of migraine equivalents, however, is recurrent vomiting. These children will complain of severe abdominal pain, usually in the middle of the abdomen, lasting several hours. The pain may be severe enough to cause the child to lie down. Loss of appetite with nausea and vomiting can occur with this pain, or separate from it. There may also be a fever, and sometimes headache pain. These bouts can last from hours to days. Physical examination reveals no other apparent reason for this "abdominal migraine."

As with other migraine symptoms, vomiting and abdominal pain are believed to be caused by changes in the brain's activity that affect the gastrointestinal tract and the centers for nausea and vomiting. These attacks of cyclical vomiting generally stop by ages five to eight and may respond well to antimigraine therapy.

MIGRAINE EQUIVALENTS AND ACTUAL MIGRAINE

How often do children go on from migraine equivalents to actual migraines? Unfortunately, the answer is: quite often—but not all the time. About 75 percent of children who experience cyclic vomiting, for instance, will go on to develop another form of migraine that includes headache pain. Generally, children who have migraine have had a higher rate of early migraine equivalents than other children—which also means that many children do not go on from migraine equivalents to later headache pain.

RESPONDING TO MIGRAINE EQUIVALENTS

Since migraine equivalents are believed to be set off by typical migraine triggers, you may actually have an opportunity to help your children develop resistance to their tendencies to migraines. To the extent that diet, exercise, and stress are implicated in migraine, developing effective ways of coping with these areas can give your child physical and emotional resources to prevent or reduce headache pain.

For example, to the extent that hypoglycemia is a cause of migraine pain, starting your children on a processed sugar–free diet will greatly reduce their susceptibility to migraine. Likewise, if either positive or negative stress triggers a migraine equivalent in your child, alternate ways of coping with stress may help the child prevent later attacks of actual migraine.

As we've said, migraine syndromes aren't "caused" by stress or diet; their source seems to be in a biochemical or nervous disorder. This disorder, however, may be no more than a tendency to translate certain dietary triggers, physical states, or emotional conditions into headache. Since diet, exercise, and emotional coping techniques can radically modify these tendencies, how much greater might their impact be if begun in childhood?

CLUSTER HEADACHES

This type of headache is rare in childhood, but it does occasionally appear. It, too, is associated with uneven blood flow. The pain is generally extremely intense, and always appears on only one side of the head, focused around the eye and the temple. The experience of the pain is as of something sharp boring into the eye. It's usually accompanied by a drooped lid, a smaller pupil, a red and tearing eye, and a stuffed and running nostril on the same side as the pain. (For more on cluster headaches, see Chapter 2.)

As opposed to the migraine child who retreats to a dark room and lies down, those with cluster headaches may frantically pace about, pushing their fist into their eye, or otherwise behaving bizarrely. Some adults with cluster have actually been known to bang their heads against the wall, as though to take their minds off the intense pain in their heads.

Cluster attacks in children usually last from twenty to forty-five minutes, rarely longer. However, the attacks may occur several times in one day, or wake the child from sleep. Cluster headaches are so named because the attacks tend to "cluster" together, perhaps in cycles of four to six weeks, as often as once a year or as infrequently as once in a lifetime. Boys are far more likely than girls to get cluster headaches, by a ratio of five or seven to one.

MIGRAINE AND EPILEPSY

Over the years, various research studies have pointed out the relationship between migraine and epilepsy. Both conditions seem to run in families, both are associated with auras, both are intermittent (that is, they express themselves as occasional "attacks," rather than as a continuous condition, such as blindness or deafness), and both may share similar triggers (for example, flashing or flickering lights). In addition, the electroencephalograms (EEGs) of migraine patients show abnormalities in brain activity, which is similar to that seen in epilepsy.

This latter indicator—abnormal brain activity—has unknown significance. It isn't clear whether abnormal EEGs in child migraineurs reflect lifelong brain patterns or simply a stage of brain development. It's possible that there is some relationship between migraine and epilepsy, but no one has yet adequately demonstrated it.

However, we do know that in some cases, child migraineurs with abnormal EEGs may benefit from antiseizure medication, treatment that is also given to epileptics. The fact that both syndromes benefit from the same medication may or may not be significant.

MUSCLE CONTRACTION HEADACHES

These used to be known as tension headaches, because they were once believed to be caused primarily by tension or other emotional factors. Now we believe that, while stress may be one trigger for this type of headache, its ultimate source is, like migraine, a neurological or biochemical disorder that originates in the brain. (For more about muscle contraction headaches, see Chapter 2.)

Some 70 percent of all children get some kind of muscle contraction headache from time to time, whatever the trigger. These are known as *acute muscle contraction headaches*, and don't require any medical intervention.

Chronic muscle contraction headaches, on the other hand, are less common in children than in adults. They bring only dull to moderate pain, but recur frequently, sometimes daily, over a period of weeks, months, or even years. The pain lasts throughout the day, experienced as a bandlike or caplike sensation squeezing the entire head. Generally, nausea and other migraine symptoms don't accompany this pain.

We still don't know just what causes this type of chronic headache pain. Despite the name, muscle contraction is not necessarily the cause. Muscle contraction may be the effect of pain—the body's braced response to an unpleasant sensation. Of course, once the head and neck muscles are contracted, their tension may make the pain worse. That's why biofeedback, which teaches people to relax certain muscles, is so often effective. Somehow, relaxing head and neck muscles helps reverse and prevent headache pain, whatever that pain's original source.

As with migraines, it's important to be clear about the

relationship of stress and other psychological factors to chronic muscle contraction headache. You may hear many people, including some doctors, suggest that your child is having tension headaches because his or her life is excessively tense. This isn't necessarily true. It's only true that your child's system is such that it translates stress—as well as some physical triggers—into headache pain. Diet and exercise may make your child less susceptible to headaches. Or your child—and your family—may need to learn some other ways of coping with or reducing stress. Perhaps your child's headaches will be the opportunity for you and your family to develop some new strengths.

RESPONDING TO YOUR CHILD'S HEADACHES: A FAMILY DYNAMIC

As we've said, migraine and muscle contraction headaches are biological disorders that can be triggered by a variety of emotional and physical causes. Once this syndrome is set into motion, it may take on a life of its own. The entire family may find itself "making use of" a child's headaches. Thus, instead of dealing directly with various stresses and conflicts within the family, a family may find itself attributing all of its problems to a sick child.

For example, if a husband and wife are in conflict about some other matter, such as someone's work schedule or someone's spending habits, they may find it easier to avoid this conflict if both are "pulling together" to respond to a child's migraines. Likewise, another child who is having difficulty at school may find it easier to complain to her parents about a little brother with a migraine than to express directly her other conflicts.

The people in these situations aren't avoiding their problems on purpose. But they may be afraid or ashamed of their real feelings, or believe that others won't respond well to them. A child's headaches may provide an opportunity to bypass issues that seem painful or difficult.

On the other hand, if one child is frequently sick, a brother or sister may respond by being "extra good" or acting like "a little grownup." The sick child may be excused from his or her share of family chores, or allowed to get out of "boring" family events, such as going to church or visiting relatives. Other children in the family may feel that they are not allowed their own share of "childish" behavior, while secretly resenting their sibling—or perhaps even blaming themselves for not being lovable enough.

These feelings may be compounded if, in addition to a headachey child, there is also an adult migraineur whose headaches require extra cooperation from the rest of the family. Those children without headaches may come to feel that being sick brings special privileges, while staying well obliges you to take on other people's burdens.

If a child in your family frequently has headaches, you might try one of the following suggestions for modifying diet, coping with menstrual migraines, or regularizing the child's schedule. If these interventions are effective, your path is clear: Help your child to understand as much as possible about what causes his or her headaches, so that s/he can continue to prevent headaches as s/he grows up.

If, however, these modifications don't work, or don't work to a great enough extent, you may want to consider behavioral and family approaches to your child's migraines. It's likely that, whatever the headaches' original cause, they have taken on a life of their own, a life that the entire family has mobilized to support. In order to treat the headaches, your child and your family may have to make some changes in behavior, so that your actions discourage headaches rather than inadvertently support them.

CHANGES IN DIET

There are a variety of foods that affect blood vessel activity and thus trigger migraines in children who are so predisposed. If your child experiences frequent migraines, we suggest that you work with a nutritionist to determine which foods are his/her triggers. Or you can try eliminating all of the foods in the following list from his or her diet. If the migraines occur less frequently or are less severe, gradually add one food per week, to see whether or not that food triggers a headache. It may be that some foods are especially upsetting to your child, while others will only trigger migraines at times that are stressful for other reasons.

FOODS THAT YOUR CHILD MAY NEED TO AVOID

chocolate
nuts
peanut butter
pork
citrus fruits
onions
pizza
sour cream
yogurt

herring
chicken livers
avocado
Nutrasweet
(aspartame)
vinegar
bananas
MSG

In addition, your child should avoid ripened cheeses, such as cheddar, Gruyère, Camembert, and Brie, although American cheese, cottage cheese, and cream cheese are permissible. Cheese spreads tend to contain additives which are not healthful for your child. Hot fresh breads, raised coffee cakes, and doughnuts contain yeast that may trigger a headache. Cola drinks and other sodas may contain preservatives, caffeine, and either natural or artificial sweeteners, all of which trigger headaches. Cured meats, such as bologna, salami, pepperoni, summer sausage, and hot dogs, often trigger headaches, as do bacon and other products that contain nitrites. Pickled, fermented, or marinated foods are other headache triggers.

Finally, many studies have suggested that migraine headaches are triggered by processed sugars, corn syrup, and other "natural" sweeteners. This research indicates that some childhood migraineurs are relatively hypoglycemic, that is, they have a tendency to produce a high level of insulin to break down their body's level of blood sugar. When they eat a food that contains processed sugar, their insulin production is stimulated even further. Apparently, there is a relation between excess insulin and catechol-amines, the substance released under stress, in the "fight or flight" reaction. In migraineurs, these catecholamines may trigger the process that leads to a headache.

Therefore, if all else fails, you might want to eliminate all processed sugar, honey, and corn syrup. That means no sugar, no sweetened cereal, no cookies, no cake, no ice cream, and no candy.

As you look at this long list of "forbidden foods," you may feel a sense of despair. "Those are all my kid's favorites!" you may be thinking. "Plus those are all normal kid foods. How can I tell my child not to eat hot dogs, dough-nuts, or pizza? How can I refuse to let my child drink Coke or hot chocolate, or forbid eating even a single candy bar?"

It isn't easy changing long-standing eating patterns, for children or for adults. But if you and your child recall the terrible distress of headache pain, making dietary changes may seem more worthwhile. Here is one suggested ap-proach to making this change:

ENLIST YOUR CHILD'S HELP IN THIS PROCESS

Explain to your child that the two of you (or three of you if two parents are available) are going to play detective. Explain that for some reason, his/her body is reacting to some foods by having a headache. You have a long list of "suspected criminals"—sugar, chocolate, hot dogs, and so on. The only way to find the "real criminals" is to conduct a scientific experiment.

Explain exactly what you plan to do: to eliminate cer-tain foods, then reintroduce them gradually, one by one. If possible, let your child help "design" the experiment, or see if s/he can figure out why eliminating and then reintrod-ucing foods will lead you to the "criminal." Emphasize that the experiment is time-limited, and give your child a cal-endar to mark off the days of the first "total elimination" month.

If you've used special foods as treats in your family, get

254 / HEADACHE RELIEF

together with your child to think up some substitute treats, either in the form of other foods or in another form entirely. The child may experience this month as difficult, but it should in no way seem like a punishment. You may want to modify the entire family's diet to some extent, or this may not be a good choice for your family. Either way, try to minimize the sense of setting the headache child apart, either through special food restrictions or through special other treats. This child *is* different and does have special needs, but neither the headache child nor the other children need to view this as "good" or "bad," as cause for special coddling or special deprivation. Perhaps you could offer other children in the family a choice between their "special" foods and the alternate treat that the child with the headache is getting.

When the time comes to reintroduce various foods, involve your child as much as possible in this process, too. Let him or her pick which foods will come back first, and in what order. Making a list of how to reintroduce foods might be a good activity during the food-free month. It will remind the child that the month won't last forever and that s/he is making at least some of the choices in this difficult situation.

When a food is reintroduced, a child could write down the name of the food on a calendar, or have you write it down. At the end of the day, you and the child can write down a few sentences about how the child feels: tired or energetic? clear thinking or confused? Focus on the positive, so that you don't "bring back" a headache by the power of suggestion! Continue with this record keeping for another five to seven days. If a child does get a headache, be sure s/he is the one to write it down, or to direct you how to write it down. Then ask, "What do you think this means about [name of new food]?" If the child is drawing his/her own conclusions about the relationship of the food to the headache, it will be much easier for him/her to give up trigger foods.

If the child wants to continue the experiment for another two or three days, go along with it. Possibly the headache was triggered by some other factor, or perhaps the child "needs" an additional headache or two to enable the giving up of a favorite food.

The more your child directs this process, the easier it will be for him/her to stick to it. After all, it's your child who will have to say "no" to cake at a friend's birthday party, or who will have to avoid buying a Coke when s/he's out with the gang. Your child should also understand that sometimes it's all right to eat a forbidden food—as long as s/he's willing to face the consequences of the headache afterwards.

To review:

1. Enlist your child's help in this process.

2. Explain exactly what you plan to do.

3. Give your child a calendar.

4. Think up some substitute treats.

5. Let him or her pick which foods will come back first. Try out each new food for five to seven days.

6. Work with the child to write down a few sentences about how s/he feels when a new food is reintroduced.

7. Ask, "What do you think this means about [name of new food]?"

DEALING WITH HORMONAL TRIGGERS

As we discussed in Chapter 8, a girl's first period often sets off a pattern of migraine that may be with her for her entire adult life. Menstrual migraine may be treated with medication, but in general, we recommend a drugless approach if at all possible, particularly for growing children.

However, a girl who tends to get headaches around the time of her period has one clear advantage in combating her migraines: She knows when to expect them. Avoiding trigger foods may be especially necessary at this time—or perhaps it is only at this time that trigger foods set a headache off. Explaining this process to your daughter and working with her to conduct her own food experiments may enable her to work out an effective headache prevention diet.

Various relaxation techniques, stretching exercises, and body awareness methods may also be helpful to your daughter, especially around the time of her period. Share the information in Chapter 6 with her, and encourage her to find a style of headache management that works for her.

Likewise, aerobic exercise seems to be helpful in preventing migraine. If your daughter is not already involved in some aerobic activity, explain that such sports as running, aerobics, basketball, hockey, skating, cross-country skiing, and bicycling help release stress and produce the endorphins that combat migraine headache. Such exercise usually needs to be practiced all month long, since the week before one's period is not a very inspiring time to begin any vigorous activity!

Children of all ages should be encouraged to take as much control as possible over their headache management. And it's doubly important for children on the brink of puberty to feel a sense of independence and responsibility. Children of this age especially need you to deal with exercise and diet in a nonpunitive way, one that allows your child to make her own use of available information about headache prevention.

"But she won't listen!" some parents may object. "She knows that eating chocolate gives her headaches, and she goes ahead and eats it anyway." Or, "I've tried to get her to exercise more, but she doesn't pay any attention."

Teenagers' stubborn insistence on doing what *we* know is bad for them is one of the most difficult parts of adolescence—at least for the adults involved! Try to remember that however painful a migraine is, it's not life threatening, nor does it involve your child in a criminal or self-destructive life-style.

Once you are convinced that your child's headaches are not from a serious cause, it is appropriate for you to refuse to allow your child's headaches to interfere with his or her household responsibilities—that is, to allow them, in every sense of the word, to be *her/his* problem. S/he should know that you are available with information and assistance, but that you will neither monitor his/her diet, nor give special privileges for getting headaches.

Then, if you still find yourself suffering in sympathy with a headache-ridden child, find some way of treating *yourself*. Get out of the house, go to a movie, lock yourself in the bathroom for a relaxing bath or shower, or pick up a favorite book. If your child's headaches don't have the power to make *you* suffer, both of you will be happier in the end.

It is possible that a child's headaches are a cry for more attention, or a sign that something is troubling him/her, either inside or outside the family. You may want to look at these issues—but consider them separately from the headaches themselves. As long as the headaches are an effective way for your child to communicate with you, s/he will have good reason to continue getting them, no matter how great the pain. Do take responsibility for your part in the communication—but leave the headaches to your child.

Finally, as we explained in Chapter 8, birth control pills and other hormone supplements are likely to make menstrual migraines worse, besides possibly putting your daughter at increased risk of stroke, heart attack, and cancer. Regardless of your own feelings about birth control and teenage sexual activity, you owe it to your child to be sure s/he has this information. Of course, no one with migraine should be using birth control pills to regularize their periods, although some doctors still prescribe them for this purpose.

REGULARIZING YOUR CHILD'S LIFE

Children with migraine or chronic headache are often sensitive to changes in their "chronobiology." That is, changes in certain biological rhythms can trigger headaches. These may include changes in bedtimes or waking times, as well as variations in mealtimes. As we explained in Chapter 7, headache sufferers often get headaches from missing or delaying meals (or from going to bed on an empty stomach), especially if they have relative hypoglycemia. Children with migraines can also get headaches from changes in weather, seasons, time zones, and altitudes.

Obviously, there is a limit to how far you can regularize your child's life. You can make sure s/he sleeps, wakes, and eats regularly. Possibly, iron supplements taken a few weeks before entering high altitudes may help prevent a migraine. Other than that, being aware of the change and avoiding other headache triggers at the same time may be the most helpful.

On the other hand, we caution against becoming overly rigid. If your child occasionally gets headaches, this is painful, but it's not a tragedy. The stress involved in panic over a schedule change may be more headache inducing than the change itself.

STRESS, THE "MIGRAINE PERSONALITY," AND THE BEHAVIORAL APPROACH TO MIGRAINE

A lot has been written about the so-called "migraine personality." This term was supposed to refer to adults whose style was rigid, perfectionistic, controlled, orderly, and meticulous, or to those who were overly fearful of making mistakes, had great need of approval from others, and experienced difficulty expressing anger. They were supposed to come from families with overly high standards of performance.

Now the medical community is rather skeptical of these typologies. People with so-called migraine personalities frequently don't have migraine, while many people with migraine don't fit the supposed personality.

Likewise, some studies have shown that children with migraine have the following personality profiles: intelligent, shy, perfectionist, sensitive, neat, easily frustrated, tense, and high-strung. Some researchers believe that the families of these children tend to have extremely high standards of performance, whether in school, sports, or some other activity, and that they discourage their children from expressing anger or other strong emotions.

Again, we don't believe it's possible to make such sweeping assumptions about child migraineurs or their families. However, since your child is having headaches, it's possible that s/he is experiencing some kinds of stress, particularly if modifying diet and other physical factors doesn't seem to be effective.

This stress may have its source in school or other places outside the family. But part of the stress may inadvertently be coming from within the family. Possibly in other families children are expressing their stress in other ways. In your family, one of your children may be signaling a problem by means of a headache.

THE BEHAVIORAL APPROACH

One way of coping with a child's headaches is a behavioral approach. This approach focuses not on analyzing underlying psychological causes, but on changing the behavior of the child and the family.

Researchers have found that once a child has a pattern of headaches, it may set up a vicious cycle. For example, the child becomes sick in school, throws up, and is embarrassed. The next day, the child is anxious about going to school, fearing the possibility of another painful migraine attack and the consequent embarrassment of being publicly sick. The stress of this fear brings on another headache. Parents and perhaps other siblings are extremely nice to the sick child, thus inadvertently reinforcing headaches as a way of getting love, attention, and other privileges.

The combination of headache-related anxiety and "rewards" for headaches may contribute to a situation where a child is almost continually missing school because of headaches. This isolates the child, possibly contributing to depression, low self-esteem, and a disabling sense of "difference as incapacity." The child never has the chance to test his or her tolerance of pain or the ability to handle the school situation, because at the first sign of a headache, he or she is staying home. This makes the school situation seem all the more frightening.

A behavioral approach focuses on getting the child back in school, with or without a headache. If the child is ten years old or older, the child and parents make a written contract that the child will attend school for one class period, with or without a headache. However, the child will attend school for no more than one class period. Thus the child is not being tested in any way ("See how long you can stay in school this week, honey").

To maximize the child's sense of responsibility, he or she is allowed to choose which period to attend, though it should be the same period each day. And a period early in the morning will cut down on the day's anxious waiting and wondering whether a headache will strike in school. At the end of a week of such attendance, the child receives a previously agreed-upon treat, such as a visit to the zoo.

During this week, the child and family agree not to discuss the child's headaches in any way. The child should be praised for attending school, but without mention of headaches, either positively or negatively. If not discussing the child's headaches at all seems too difficult, the parents may ask the child about them at two regularly scheduled times, during which the child describes the nature and degree of the headache, if any, and the parents express recognition of the child's situation and their belief that it will eventually improve. (For the child of eight years and under, further involvement and discussion may be necessary.)

Part of the family contract includes an agreement that the child will not discuss the headaches with anyone except the parents, and will respond, "I'd rather not talk about it," if anyone asks. This gives the child a clear plan to stick to, and again reduces the attention on the headache.

Gradually, the number of periods the child attends can be increased, as the child learns to focus on what can be done in spite of the headaches, rather than to fear the possibility of an attack. Not only should school attendance increase with this plan, but the number of the child's headaches should decrease, especially if diet and exercise suggestions are also being followed.

FAMILY THERAPY

If the other approaches in this chapter don't work—or even if they do—a family with a headache-ridden member may want to consider family counseling. In family counseling, the family meets as a group with a trained professional, who encourages family members to express their feelings and to work out new ways of dealing with one another.

Family counseling may be helpful for a number of reasons. Regardless of the sources of a headache, a sick child affects a family. Both children and adults may need to work out their feelings and to find out directly how other family members are feeling. The child with the headache may feel guilty or worried about the strain s/he imagines s/he is putting on the rest of the family. Siblings, or even parents, may feel some anger, resentment, or guilt about the child's headaches and their consequences.

Family counseling will be even more helpful if family issues are part of the stress that provokes a child's headaches. As we've said before, every family has stress, just like every person does. Headaches may be the place where your family's stress shows up, just as other families' stress shows up in their own ways. They may even end up working to your family's advantage: By dealing with the problems the headache is expressing, your family may work out issues that it could otherwise sweep under the rug.

BIOFEEDBACK FOR CHILDREN

One of the most effective treatments for headache in children is biofeedback training (for more on this training, see Chapter 4). Children have the advantage of being young enough to learn quickly; they get involved in the process; they practice it; and as a result, they learn these techniques effectively. A very high percentage of children improve with biofeedback training, no matter what the diagnosis of the root causes of their headaches.

HEADACHE MEDICATION FOR CHILDREN

Normally, we don't recommend medication for headaches in the very young. However, sometimes occasional symptomatic medication for migraine (controlling pain or blood vessel activity) is the best way of dealing with the headache in the short run, while longer-range solutions are also being sought. In some situations, a daily preventive medicine is the best treatment. Here are the types of medication we use for children:

ANALGESICS

Off-the-shelf pain relievers like salicylates (aspirin), acetaminophen (Tylenol, Datril), and ibuprofen (Advil, Nuprin) are used for one-time acute headache attacks. Generally, Tylenol is the drug of choice for children, when it works, since aspirin has been implicated in a childhood disease known as Reyes' syndrome and ibuprofen's effects on children have not yet been sufficiently studied. However, aspirin may work better than Tylenol on certain children.

As in adults, analgesics in children can produce a rebound effect, wherein, the more often these painkillers are taken, the more the child comes to depend upon them. Eventually, these painkillers end up making a child's headaches worse, and must be discontinued. The best way to avoid this situation is for you or your child to document on a headache calendar when analgesics are used. If they are used more than three days per week, you should inform your physician. (For more information on the rebound effect, see Chapter 3.)

Stronger symptomatic medications include the combination drugs isometheptene mucate (Midrin) and ergotamine tartrate (Cafergot), which both contain vasoconstrictors that shrink dilated blood vessels. Preventive medicines include the antihistamine cyproheptadine (Periactin), which is particularly effective for children, as well as antidepressants, beta blockers, and calcium channel blockers. (For more on these different types of medication, see Chapter 3.)

Migraines that are associated with vomiting may be treated with antinausea medication such as promethazine HCl (Phenergan). This may be administered orally or by rectal suppository.

Sometimes, antinausea medication helps the child enough so that she or he is able to sleep. If not, you might follow up twenty to thirty minutes later with isomethep-tene mucate or ergotamine tartrate, as mentioned above.

We've found that the need for children's preventive medication is reduced significantly around the summer as school pressures are reduced. We often find it useful to discontinue medication over the summer, and then recon-sider whether to start it up again in the fall.

As with adult headaches, we don't expect medication to cure them, since we still don't understand their under-lying cause. What we do expect is to reduce headache fre-quency by 80 percent. It's also important to remember that headache syndromes in children sometimes cure them-selves spontaneously. This seems especially likely to us if positive changes are made in diet, exercise, and family pat-terns.

APPENDIX

PSYCHOPHYSIOLOGICAL EVALUATION

THIS PROCEDURE COLLECTS DATA on important physiological activity related to muscle activity in (1) the head and neck and (2) skin temperature (which tells us something about blood vessel activity). Both of these are important in headache disorders.

A variety of stimuli are presented to the patient and reactions are monitored: is the patient more muscularly reactive, that is, do her muscles tense when stressed; vascularly reactive, do her hands get cold when stressed, or both. This can be helpful in diagnosis and patient education.

We also explore psychological issues related to family relationships and stress, to determine if they affect the headache syndrome in any way.

DEBRIEFING LOG

The debriefing log that we use aids in compliance with behavioral exercises; it is used by patients between sessions to document home practice, biofeedback, relaxations using tapes, written instructions, etc. It helps patients to record their progress and evaluate the effect of practice sessions on headache.

The Log indicates to the patient and doctor that decreased tension is connected to a decrease in head pain. It helps a patient get more in touch with what it *feels* like to be relaxed, (e.g., warm, calm, etc.).

Some patients have trouble completing the Log because they do not take the time.

CALENDARS

The headache calendar is one of the most important aspects of our program because it is the most accurate way of recording data and monitoring progress. Self-reporting is generally inaccurate and inadequate.

Patients are instructed to fill in severity of headache by number (see top right of page) and duration by recording headache activity during the day. For example, a mild headache in the afternoon of the second day of the month would be signified by the number 1 in the second box.

On the fourteenth day, the number 3 signifies an incapacitating headache, lasting all day on day one of her period. She used two Cafergot tablets, obtained moderate relief (indicated by the number 2 in the Relief box). The headache may have additionally been triggered by red wine (see Trigger box).

The calendars are initially filled out by the doctor or nurse with the patient. With the aid of the calendars, patients are instructed on appropriate use of preventive and symptomatic medications used at the time of the headache, to aid in increasing proper use, and minimizing misuse.

PSYCHOPHYSIOLOGICAL
EVALUATION

(Used for interviewing prior to biofeedback session)

I. REVIEW OF HEADACHE SYMPTOMS
AND MEDICATIONS
   A. Any environmental precipitants for onset and/or increase in frequency?

   B. Does the patient see stress as related to headaches?

   C. Has the patient taken any of these medications previously?
      1. Wigraine
      2. Cafergot
      3. Midrin
      4. Periactin
      5. Phenergan
      6. Elavil (amitriptyline HCl)

II. FAMILY HISTORY
   A. Relationship problems (i.e., with spouse, children, parents, etc.)?

   B. Lingering grief reaction to family member's death?

C. Family members' perceptions of patient's headaches (e.g., sympathetic, viewed as malingering, viewed as psychological problem)

D. Family (and personal) history of alcohol/drug abuse?

E. Family (and personal) history of psychological treatment or issues?

III. VOCATIONAL PROBLEMS?
A. Stress on job with workers or superiors

B. Compensation

C. Hours

D. Environment—odors, pollutants, noise

IV. SOCIAL PROBLEMS (INVOLVEMENT WITH OTHER PEOPLE, ETC.)?
A. Interpersonal relationships

B. Shyness

C. Getting along with others

V. HABITS

A. Pleasurable activities (leisure-time activities, hobbies, interests, time for *self*)?

B. Exercise? How frequently do you exercise? Which forms of exercise do you do regularly?

C. Recreational drug usage (now and in the past)?

D. DFA? Difficulty falling asleep? How many minutes?

E. EMA? Early morning awakening? What time?

F. Rested in A.M.?

G. Constipation?

H. Appetite problems/weight changes?

I. Sexual problems (e.g., decreased frequency/physical problems)?

J. Concentration/memory problems?

K. Bruxism/clenching?

L. TMJ (pain or clicking on opening mouth, clenching or chewing)?

M. Cervical tightness? Do you rub your neck a lot during the day?

N. Cold extremities? Does your spouse complain about your cold feet?

VI. SELF-REPORT
A. Does patient view self as "nervous?"

B. Does patient view self as "being depressed?"

C. Does patient view self as being able to relax?

D. Previous biofeedback/relaxation training?

VII. ANYTHING ELSE THAT PATIENT CAN ADD RE: HEADACHE HISTORY?

IMPRESSION: TREATMENT:

Reference: Randall Weeks, Ph.D., and Stephen Baskin, Ph.D., Directors, New England Institute of Behavioral Medicine, Stamford, CT 06902.

DEBRIEFING LOG

(Used by patients between sessions with biofeedback technician)

BODY AWARENESS

DATE/ TIME	LEVEL OF TENSION[1]		HEADACHE LEVEL[2]		DURING THE EXERCISE		QUESTIONS FOR THE DOCTOR
	BEFORE EXERCISE	AFTER EXERCISE	BEFORE EXERCISE	AFTER EXERCISE	BODY SENSATIONS[3]	DIFFICULTIES[4]	

KEY:

[1] Totally relaxed 1 2 3 4 5 6 7 8 9 10 Extremely tense

[2] 0 = no headache   1 = mild   2 = moderate/severe   3 = incapacitating pain

[3] Heaviness, lightness, tingling, etc.

[4] Mind wandering, interruptions, areas difficult to relax (shoulders, face, etc.)

THE NEW ENGLAND CENTER FOR HEADACHE
HEADACHE CALENDAR

Name

	01	02	03	04	05	06	07	08	09	10	11	12	13	14
Morning														
Afternoon														
Evening														
Sleeptime														
Medication														
_____														
_____														
_____														
_____														
_____														

Relief   0-1-2-3   (0)-NONE, (1)-slight relief, (2)-Moderate

TRIGGERS:

Periods:

#1 Mild Headache
#2 Moderate-Severe
#3 Incapacitating

Month   Year

| 15 | 16 | 17 | 18 | 19 | 20 | 21 | 22 | 23 | 24 | 25 | 26 | 27 | 28 | 29 | 30 | 31 |

relief, (3)-complete relief

MIGRAINE DIET

This diet includes all the known triggers for headache. This does not mean that each of these will serve as a trigger for any one individual. Patients are asked to eliminate all potential trigger foods—and should reintroduce them one at a time to evaluate their individual effect.

FOOD GROUP	FOODS ALLOWED	FOODS TO AVOID
Eggs	Limit intake to 3 times per week (for cholesterol reasons).	Raw eggs.
Potatoes & Substitutes	White, sweet potato, pasta, and rice.	None.
Vegetables	All fresh, frozen, canned, or dried (except those not allowed) & vegetable juices. Limit tomatoes to ½ cup daily. Also allowed: Asparagus, broccoli, beets, carrots, corn, lettuce, greens, squash, pumpkin & zucchini.	Beans (lima, Italian, pole, broad, fava, navy, pinto, garbanzo, lentils, string, snow peas), chile peppers, pickles, olives.
Fruits	Fresh, frozen, or canned fruits or juices (e.g., prunes, apples, applesauce, cherries, apricots, peaches, pears, fruit cocktail). ½ cup/day limit: orange, grapefruit, tangerine, pineapple, lemon, lime. ½ per day: banana.	Fermented dry fruits (raisins, figs, etc.), avocado, banana peel extract, red plums, papaya & passion fruit.
Soups	Cream soups made from allowed foods, homemade broths.	Commercial canned soups, bouillon cubes, soups made from beer, cheese, beans, soup cubes, or meat extracts. Soup base with yeast or MSG.

(continued)

FOOD GROUP	FOODS ALLOWED	FOODS TO AVOID
Desserts & Sweets	Cakes, cookies made without chocolate, small amounts of yeast or vanilla, gelatin, sherbet, puddings (made with skim milk). Sugar, honey, jam, jelly, hard candy & syrup.	Cheese-filled desserts, cakes/ cookies made with chocolate, large amounts of vanilla or yeast. Desserts containing dried fermented fruits (e.g., mincemeat pie), pineapple, raspberries, banana, or yogurt. Candy made from chocolate, carob, or licorice. Ice cream, pudding (made with whole milk), chocolate syrup.
Beverages	Decaffeinated coffee, tea, sodas (7-Up, ginger ale, decaf colas, club soda) & fruit juices. Limit caffeine sources to 2 cups per day (regular coffee, teas & cola).	All beer, alcohol & wine (especially Chianti, sherry, sauterne, Riesling), chocolate, cocoa.
Milk/ Dairy Products	Milk, homogenized 1% or skim. Cheese: American, cottage, rogatio, cream, Velveeta, pot, and farmer. Limit yogurt to ½ cup per day (skim milk based).	Cultured dairy products, sour cream, buttermilk, chocolate milk, acidophilus milk. Aged cheese: boursault, brick, Brie, bleu, Colby, Camembert, cheddar, Gouda, Gruyère, mozzarella, Parmesan, Emmentaler, provolone, Romano, Roquefort, Stilton.
Bread/ Cereal	Commercial breads: enriched white, wheat, rye, French, Italian, bagels, English muffin, melba toast, crackers & quick breads. All hot & dry cereals.	Hot, fresh homemade yeast breads, cheese breads, or crackers. Fresh yeast coffee cake, doughnuts, sourdough bread. Any product containing nuts, chocolate, or banana peel extracts. Cereals to which brewer's yeast has been added. Minimize use of cereals/breads containing chocolate, dried fruits, pineapple, raspberries, banana.

FOOD GROUP	FOODS ALLOWED	FOODS TO AVOID
Meat, Fish, Poultry	All fresh or frozen beef, veal, fish, poultry, lamb & pork. Tuna (water packed).	Aged, canned, cured, or processed meats or game. Chicken & kidney organ meats, beef liver, salted or dried fish (caplin, herring, cod), hot dogs, bologna, fermented sausage (e.g., salami, pepperoni, summer sausage), bacon, meat prepared with papaya and other meat tenderizers (Accent, MSG), caviar, or peanut butter.
Fats	Butter, margarine, cooking oil, whipped cream, and all except those which are fermented.	Sour cream.
Misc.	Salt, lemon juice, white vinegar, pepper, herbs, spices, fresh homemade gravy.	Brewer's yeast, yeast concentrate & products made with brewer's yeast, yeast extracts (e.g., mormite, bovri, MSG, soy sauce, all aged & fermented products). Meat tenderizer, seasoned salt, pizza & cheese sauce. Any pickled, preserved, or marinated food, commercial gravies, mixed dishes (e.g., cheese blintzes, lasagna, macaroni & cheese, & TV dinners). Nuts, seeds (e.g., sesame, sunflower & pumpkin), peanut butter & peanuts.

INDEX

creative visualization in, 30–
31, 35, 44, 132, 135, 154,
157–60, 172
deep, 123–25, 126, 127,
150–51, 171
guided, 154
meditation in, 33, 124, 125,
132, 161–62, 229
by the numbers, 154–55
overall body, 153–54
passive, 132
progressive, 132, 144, 153
REM ("rapid eye movement")
sleep, 71–72, 75, 77
Reyes' syndrome, 262
Rosum, Robert W., 95

saccharin, 197
salicin, 99
salt, 203, 218, 244
scotoma, 62, 243
secondary gains, 164, 165–68,
259
sedatives, 102, 104, 105, 108,
119
Selye, Hans, 149
serotonergic system, 52
serotonin, 17–18, 26, 70, 92,
111, 112, 114, 118, 126,
142
migraines and, 59, 60–61,
64, 221
sex headaches, 82
shoulders, 46–47, 53, 63, 72,
133, 137, 175
sinuses, 23, 27, 48, 58, 80, 190,
191, 213, 236
sinus headaches, 28, 74, 79–
80, 102, 236
off-the-shelf medication for,
102–3, 115, 205–6
skin, 63, 78, 213, 218, 224
sleep, 61, 111, 150, 182, 243,
244
caffeine and, 207, 208

changes in, 66, 70, 71–72,
209
disturbances of, 18, 51, 52,
71, 73, 77, 83, 207, 238,
246
headache from, 51, 53–54,
57, 68, 71, 72, 75, 208, 236,
238
REM, 71–72, 75, 77
smoking, 30, 37, 77, 117, 185,
187, 190, 193, 200, 204–5,
223, 225
sonophobia, 57, 64, 217, 243
spinal cord, 24–25, 27, 55, 126
steroids, 66, 70, 71, 104, 116,
197
stress, 13, 14, 26, 30, 52, 80,
113, 129, 140, 148–50,
212, 226, 241
biological basis of, 149–50
in children, 244, 247, 250,
258, 259–61
"fight or flight" response in,
52–53, 62, 128, 138, 149,
193, 194, 206, 253
in menstrual migraines, 66,
69, 226
in migraines, 57, 66, 67, 69, 92
in muscle contraction
headaches, 50–54
see also emotions; relaxation
stroke, 63, 87, 101, 102, 204,
223, 225
subdural hematoma, 84–85
suboccipital ice pillow (S.I.P.),
172
substance abuse, 73, 91, 105
sugar, 12, 64, 69, 186, 190, 192,
194–95, 198, 201, 206,
211, 219, 252–53
blood, see blood sugar
sulfisoxazole, 197
surgery, 31, 48, 112, 117, 118
sympathetic nervous system,
128, 150